T0271544

HOW TO GO
VEGAN

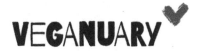

VEGANUARY

HOW TO GO
VEGAN

**The why, the how, and everything
you need to make going vegan easy**

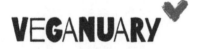

HODDER &
STOUGHTON

First published in Great Britain in 2017 by Hodder & Stoughton
An Hachette UK company

This edition published in 2021

1

Copyright © Veganuary 2017

A CIP catalogue record for this title is available from the British Library

Hardback ISBN 9781529368871
Ebook 9781473680975

Typeset in Celeste 11/15.5 pt by
Palimpsest Book Production Limited, Falkirk, Stirlingshire

Printed and bound in Great Britain by Clays Ltd, Elcograf S.p.A.

Hodder & Stoughton policy is to use papers that are natural,
renewable and recyclable products and made from wood grown in sustainable
forests. The logging and manufacturing processes are expected to conform to
the environmental regulations of the country of origin.

Hodder & Stoughton Ltd
Carmelite House
50 Victoria Embankment
London EC4Y 0DZ

www.hodder.co.uk

CONTENTS

FOREWORD

By Evanna Lynch,
actress and Veganuary Ambassador

Whether you are already vegan, vegetarian, pescatarian, flexitarian, v-curious or you're just contemplating making changes to your diet, then you've already made one huge leap on your journey – you're reading this book! Simply by setting the intention to learn about living a cruelty-free life I believe you are vegan at heart, which is the first bold step to being vegan in practice.

In a way, veganism is not such a radical change; it can be more like a return to self and simply aligning your practices with your principles. Most of us are not brought up or socially conditioned to choose the vegan option, and yet most of us would agree we want to live a life that doesn't cause unnecessary suffering to other living beings. Going vegan, I felt like I was becoming more myself and very quickly felt more comfortable in my skin. It's exciting to uncover another piece of your identity, liberating in fact. Veganism was a big piece of the puzzle for me, and it might be for you too. But while recognising that I was against animal cruelty in any form was one thing, actually becoming vegan took some time, patience, research and, most of all, community with other vegans. I read *Eating Animals* by Jonathan Safran Foer and felt thoroughly well-versed in the reasons why I was now vegan, and riled up to revamp my whole life. But I forgot to account for the fact that I was unlearning two decades' worth of living a completely different lifestyle, and that there was a method to making going vegan easier. I quickly learned that going vegan required compassion for myself as much as for the animals. I urge you to be gentle with yourself as you work towards integrating veganism seamlessly into your life. I wish I could have followed up *Eating Animals* with this beautiful, inspiring, information-packed tome you're reading, which feels like a friendly vegan fairy godmother taking your hand and guiding you down your personal, tailor-made path to becoming the best vegan you can be. *How to Go Vegan* is a fantastic introduction to all of the reasons why you might want to give veganism a go, how you can live it, and will be something you can go back to again and again, and share with your sceptical mother and curious cousin alike. One thing I'd like to imprint on your brain is that veganism is not about being perfect. And it isn't about rules and restrictions; it is about living with compassion and mindfulness – for animals, for yourself, for other humans, for our planet. You will struggle, you may make mistakes, you might feel like you're being awkward, but you'll learn that there's no such thing as a perfect vegan. You may even be tentative about sharing your new vegan life or using the V word at all because you're afraid of facing judgement, as I was. But once you do 'come out' as vegan you'll find that the vegan community is incredibly loving and supportive, friendly and thoughtful, and they make the sassiest memes. You'll find that people are just as pleased that you want to help save animals' lives and the planet, and they're eager to help you on your journey. So talk to people and find your mentors and role models in the community – your vibe attracts your tribe, as they say! Most of all, just focus on doing your personal best from day to day.

The best piece of advice I got as a new vegan was to introduce delicious new vegan foods to my diet before cutting things out – to make my vegan life feel joyful and abundant – and I believe that is the way to make it sustainable. So start to try different plant milks and meat replacements alongside what you would normally eat, until they become your everyday norm, and the meat, eggs and dairy can fall out of your life without leaving a huge hungry hole behind. If you immerse yourself in all these new delicious vegan foods (and make a point to treat yo'self often), then it won't feel like you are depriving yourself of anything – instead you've opened up a whole new world of options. Yes, it will be an adjustment and you may find yourself causing a traffic jam in the vegetable aisle of your grocery store googling the difference between a yam and a sweet potato (helpful tip: nobody really knows the difference but they are closely related cousins in the root vegetable family), but you've got this book, and you've also got the benefit of the collective wisdom and experience of the Veganuary team right here in front of you, and believe me, they know what they're talking about.

And when you hear people saying that vegans are 'extreme' and it's a lifestyle of sacrifice remember that the opposite is in fact true – it's about celebrating food and life! It really is a beautiful lifestyle and I trust when you fully dive in you will fall in love with it, as I have. This book is a great first step. I think you'll find that it helps to demystify veganism and show you that it's not that complicated after all. Veganuary are doing amazing work helping people give veganism a try for a month, and whatever your goals are, I think you'll find that you are happier, healthier and more content with yourself than ever before. With lots of love and good vibes to you as you embark on your vegan journey!

Evanna xox

INTRODUCTION

You've bought this book – or been given it – because you're the kind of person who cares about something. It might be animal welfare, the environment or world hunger. It could be water shortages, land degradation or deforestation. Or perhaps your concerns relate to climate change, loss of wild-life, antibiotic resistance, pollution or looking after your own health. If you care about any of these things – *and who doesn't?* – then it's natural you would want to do your bit, to make choices that don't create greater suffering in the world and to protect our planet.

It's easy to feel helpless in the face of global problems. We may think we can have no impact no matter what we do, and that these issues require national governments and inter-national partnerships to find solutions. We may think that one person, one ordinary person, can't make a difference. But we'd be wrong. There is something all of us can do that helps ease the burden on the planet, promotes well-being, protects wildlife and aids the world's poorest, and we can do it three times a day. Every day. It is, of course, our food choices.

What we choose to buy, cook and eat has consequences that extend way beyond our taste buds and bellies. The breakfast bacon may have come from a factory-farmed pig whose feed was grown on land where ancient rainforests once stood, who was fed antibiotics routinely just to keep him alive and whose meat, when processed, is known to cause bowel cancer in people. Or what about the milk in our tea? It may have come from a cow who lived her whole life in a shed, who was fed grain that could have instead been used to feed the world's most hungry and whose slurry contributes significantly to climate change and water pollution.

We're not told these things on the label but it doesn't make them any less true.

As the full impact of animal agriculture on our world becomes clearer, more and more people are choosing to avoid eating animal products altogether. They may call themselves 'vegan' or 'plant-based', or they may not choose a label at all, but the number of people who avoid meat, milk and eggs is rising exponentially, and this is happening all around the world.

Since 2004, the number of vegans in the United States has risen from 290,000 to 9.7 million – a rise of more than 3,000 per cent.[1] In the United Kingdom, in just five years, to 2019, the number of vegans was estimated to have grown from 150,000 to 600,000[2]. Veganism is growing so fast that these statistics are out of date almost as soon as they are published.

Unsurprisingly, the range of vegan foods available has skyrocketed to meet this booming market. In the US, retail sales of plant-based foods grew by more than 11 per cent in 2019,[3] while in the UK, the number of new trademarks registered for vegan food and drink products continues its upward trajectory.[4] It's a trend that is happening all over the world.

All this delicious, readily available food makes it even easier for people to choose animal-free products, and this helps create more vegans, who then demand more delicious vegan products, and that creates even more vegans. You see the pattern? This is a movement with powerful momentum behind it. In fact, it appears to be unstoppable.

Perhaps you're already vegan, vegetarian or v-curious, or you've tried being vegan and fallen off the wagon. Maybe you have friends and family who are vegan or interested in giving it a go. This book is for you. We don't ask for perfection, or for you to make yourself miserable by putting too much pressure on yourself. It's OK to make mistakes and have the odd slip-up. Most vegans did exactly the same when they started out, too.

WHAT EXACTLY *IS* A VEGAN?

Vegans eat no animal products at all, from the obvious items like meat, milk and eggs to the less obvious like honey. This book focuses on the foods that we eat, but most vegans will also avoid wearing animal products like fur, leather, silk and wool, and will also choose household products and cosmetics that contain no animal-derived ingredients.

We hope this book, which is intended as a practical guide to introduce you to plant-based eating, will help you on your way. Read it from cover to cover or just dip in as you wish. In it, we explain not just *why* we should embrace a plant-based diet – for animals, health and the environment – but *how* that can be done. We take the mystery out of where to shop, what to buy and how to keep eating the foods you love. We discuss nutrition and pass on our top tips for making sure you get everything you need from the foods you eat. We reveal the animal ingredients that can sneak into the foods you buy, and give you some great meal plans to get you started. We give you the support you need to try vegan for a month, from getting started on Day 1 to what you might decide to do on Day 32. And we talk you through how to deal with questions from family and friends, advise on how to travel as a vegan, reassure you about bringing up vegan children and offer our top choices for further reading and viewing.

WHAT IS VEGANUARY?

Veganuary is a UK charity with global reach that encourages people around the world to try vegan for a month in January or anytime in the year, alongside hundreds of thousands of others. We offer free support and advice and a non-judgemental approach for everyone who registers to take part at veganuary.com.

'For me it took 38 years to be ready to make that full commitment, and some people may never get to that stage, but Veganuary is a great opportunity to try it out. I genuinely think that for a lot of people, it will be much easier than they would have anticipated. They'll feel different, they'll have more energy and they'll just feel cleaner.'

Jasmine Harman, television presenter, UK, Veganuary Class of 2014 and Veganuary Ambassador

WHY TRY VEGAN?

• • •

While this book is all about the *how*, we actually need to begin by talking about the *why*. These are the reasons that most people give for trying vegan in the first place, and they are also what motivates them to stick with it in the face of difficult questions, mocking friends or a poor food offering when eating out. Knowing your own personal *why* is fundamental to the *how*.

There are lots of reasons why people try vegan for 31 days – animals, the environment, sustainability, world hunger, personal health, faith, global human health or just because it's a new challenge.

Whatever the reason that prompts someone to try plant-based eating in the first place, it often becomes just one of many good reasons why they choose to stick with it in the long term. For example, someone may try vegan to see how it boosts their athletic performance but along the way find out how chickens are factory farmed, and this becomes another motivating factor. Another person may cut out animal products because they learn that male calves are killed by

3

the dairy industry but they stay vegan because they find out more about that industry's contribution to climate change. Everyone's journey is different, and all reasons are equally valid.

'This was just the right path for me. I felt like as soon as I went vegan, I was more myself, like I was just living according to what I believed, which is such a freeing thing once you finally commit to it.'
Evanna Lynch, actress, UK, Veganuary Ambassador

But the top reason people give – the reason that most people say motivated them to try vegan – is to end animal suffering.

'All through my life I'd wanted to be vegan (for the animals), but for one reason or another I was daunted by it so put off making any change. When I heard about Veganuary, it was a perfect opportunity to make the change I really wanted and try again. What made it work this time is the world is a changed place; there is so much variety and so many options out there that the transition was simple and there is not a single thing I feel I miss out on.'
Julia B. Kent, UK, Class of 2019

WHY TRY VEGAN? –
YOUR TWO-MINUTE GUIDE

If you're short of time and keen to get to the 'how' as quickly as possible, this is your two-minute guide to all the reasons why people try vegan. Once you've read it, you may want to jump straight into the practical tips and get started. That's fine. Go right ahead and turn to page 67 – or you may prefer to read a little more about any or all of the reasons. It's your call. Whatever you choose, you might like to revisit this *why* section later on to refresh your knowledge or if you feel as though your motivation is flagging.

ANIMALS

This is the number one reason why people go vegan. It's obvious that animals must die for people to eat meat, but most people are shocked to learn that animals are killed in the egg and dairy industries, too. Male calves are often unwanted by-products of the dairy industry, and billions of day-old chicks are killed because they are the wrong sex to lay eggs. Did you know that most chickens and pigs are still intensively farmed, and that there are no welfare laws governing the slaughter of fish at sea?

'I don't really know what I expected of this 'experiment', but I certainly didn't expect this sense of relief I'm feeling. Relief that I've finally gone vegan and listened to that little voice inside that told me this is the right thing to do. Relief that I've opted out of the system that abuses and kills animals. Relief that my ideals and actions are now in line with each other. I'm just so happy I'm doing this. Two days before the New Year, I was talking with a vegan friend who told me about Veganuary and I joined on a whim. And now I'm not going back!

Ennys F. Aberystwyth, UK,
Class of 2021

ENVIRONMENT

Eating animal products is one of the top four ways each of us contributes to climate-changing emissions, along with driving cars, flying and having children.[1] The great news is that we can help protect the planet with every plant-based meal we eat. Since producing vegan foods also requires less land and water than producing animal products, being vegan is also how we can protect forests, hedgerows, waterways and all the world's other wild places and their inhabitants.

WORLD HUNGER

What we choose to eat has an impact on people all over the world. Currently, we produce more than enough food for everyone on the planet, but still one billion people go hungry every day. War, poverty and natural disasters all play a part, but so too does the fact that we feed so much of the world's cereal and soya harvest to farmed animals instead of to people. More than 96 per cent of the protein fed to cows is lost in the conversion from animal feed to meat, more than 90 per cent for pork, 80 per cent for poultry and 75 per cent for milk and eggs.[2] What a waste!

PERSONAL HEALTH

People often report that their skin, hair, sinuses, digestion and sleep improve after eating vegan foods for 31 days. Others say they have more energy, better mental clarity and their sporting performance improves. Some have told us that their chronic fatigue symptoms have reduced and that their depression symptoms were relieved. In the long term, eating a plant-based diet can also reduce the risk of high blood pressure, heart disease, type 2 diabetes and some cancers. Great news all round!

'Veganism has changed my life in so many ways. It changed the way I physically feel. I didn't realise how tired and bloated I felt all the time until I stopped eating meat. My skin is clear and smoother, my digestion has improved and my anxiety has significantly decreased.'

Julie M., Arizona, USA,
Veganuary Class of 2017

GLOBAL HEALTH

Farming animals has the potential to affect huge swathes of the global population. Many of the diseases that harm and kill people started out in farmed animals, and three quarters of all emerging infectious diseases in people have come from animals. Covid-19 is one example of how viruses can transmit from animals when people harm and exploit them. Avian flu is another example, and the H5N1 type has a mortality rate in people of 60 per cent.[3] Meanwhile, the vast amounts of antibiotics we use to keep farmed animals alive have contributed to the emergence of antibiotic-resistant superbugs, and this also threatens people worldwide.

FAITH

Increasingly, people of different faiths are embracing veganism as a way of living that is consistent with their own beliefs. At the core of many faiths lie teachings of compassion, equity, love and respect – all of which are at the heart of veganism, too. For others who do not follow an organised religion, becoming vegan may just sit better with their own spirituality, helping them connect to something deeper (call it what you will!), and putting into practice their own compassionate values.

ADVENTURE

Some people undertake 31 days of vegan eating because of the challenge of trying something different. Maybe they want to experience new ways of shopping, cooking and eating because they're stuck in a culinary rut. Perhaps they feel their health needs a bit of a boost. They may not have any preconceived ideas about what being vegan will do for them, but they try it just because.

> 'Best. Decision. Ever!'
>
> *Albie J., London, UK, Veganuary Class of 2017*

Whatever your reason for trying vegan: we wish you the best of luck. This book is here to help you.

FOR ANIMALS

'It was such a good decision! I no longer feel guilty
about what I eat – my diet now aligns with my beliefs
that animals aren't for us to use, and that we are all
equal.'

Lana M., Auckland, New Zealand,
Veganuary Class of 2017

From the invasive process of artificial insemination to
gassing newborn male chicks and surgery without pain relief,
farmed animals suffer the world over for their meat, milk
and eggs.

Most meat – including 95 per cent of the chicken sold in
the UK[1] and more than 99 per cent in the US[2] – comes from
animals who have been intensively reared. They are kept in
cages and pens, or crammed inside immense barns with tens
of thousands of other animals. It is impossible for farmers
to check every individual chicken, duck or turkey each day,

and so the sick and injured are often simply left to die.

Some countries do have higher welfare standards than others. Switzerland, for example, has banned the cages known as 'farrowing crates', where pigs are confined to give birth. In Sweden, all pigs must have straw. These, though, are exceptions. In most other countries – including the UK, Canada, USA and Australia – many hens farmed for eggs are still held in cages, mother pigs can be kept in crates for prolonged periods and straw for bedding and rooting is often denied. It's easy to forget that every one of the billions of farmed animals in the world is an individual who forms friendship bonds, has preferences and displays a distinct character. To truly understand this, we'd recommend a visit to your nearest farmed-animal sanctuary to meet the rescued cows, pigs and chickens. Not only is this one of the most uplifting experiences you will ever have, it also removes all doubt about there being two different kinds of animals: those with whom we share our homes, and those whom we eat. At sanctuaries like The Retreat (UK), Edgar's Mission (Australia) and Catskill Animal Sanctuary and Animal Place (both in the US), this distinction breaks down, and you will see that the sheep in the field isn't really so different from the dog on your sofa. Both like a belly rub and will steal your sandwiches when you're not looking!

Deep down, many of us may have an uneasy feeling that there is something not quite right with eating meat, but we try to take comfort in the notion that farmed animals have a good life and a humane death. We're sorry, but this just isn't the case. Difficult as this section on animals is to read, we urge you to give it a try. After all, the suffering of animals is the leading reason why people choose to become vegan. So, read on, and we promise that things will lighten up again in the next section. Take a deep breath. Ready?

CHICKENS

Anyone who's ever met a chicken will know what huge characters they can be. They are active, inquisitive and love to root around, foraging and exploring. They dustbathe and preen to keep their skin and feathers in tip-top shape, and love to sunbathe – lying on their sides, wings outstretched, eyes closed.

For farmed chickens, whether they are reared for meat or for their eggs, none of this is possible.

Almost all chickens reared for meat are kept inside huge warehouse-style hangars with tens of thousands of other birds. Because they have been bred to grow as big as possible as quickly as possible, their bodies outgrow their bone strength and their legs may break beneath them. Those who cannot stand up suffer skin burns from the ammonia in the litter that covers the floor. Their hearts cannot cope with their ballooning weight, and heart failure is all too common. The dead may be taken away, or just left to rot among the living birds.

Hens reared for their eggs scarcely get a better time of it. Most spend their whole reproductive lives in cages, even across the European Union where battery cages were banned in 2012. When that law was brought in, the industry could have moved to free-range systems, but instead it simply lobbied for bigger cages. And it won. The new 'improved' colony cages have a perch and a scratch pad and are big enough to house 80 birds – but they are still cages. Where the original battery cages allowed each hen space the size of an A4 sheet of paper (which is just a little larger than letter-sized paper in Canada and the US), the additional space in the colony cages is less than the size of one beer mat per hen.[3]

In the US, 75 per cent of hens are held in cages[4] while in Australia, more than half of the country's flock are also caged.[5] None of these birds are able to express their natural behaviours, such as nesting, foraging and dustbathing. It's not just a denial of their instincts that causes so much suffering; the industry takes active measures to push the birds to their biological limits, no matter the toll it takes on their bodies. After all, this is a business which aims to maximise profits, so artificial lights are switched on for prolonged periods to encourage the birds to lay even more eggs. A lot of calcium is required to make all those eggshells, and the mineral is taken from the birds' bones, which leads to the well-documented 'extremely high frequency and severity of damage' to their bones.[6] It's a price the industry is willing to pay for plentiful eggs.

These birds might naturally live ten years or more, but by the age of 18 months they are past their productive peak, and there is no happy retirement. They are loaded into crates and shipped to slaughterhouses, where they are killed and their scrawny, broken-down bodies either sent to land-fill sites or turned into processed products such as pies, soups and nuggets. Poultry is specifically excluded from the Humane Methods of Slaughter Act in the US, so there are no federal laws to protect them from suffering at slaughter there.[7]

The hens themselves are not the only victims of the egg industry. With such a high turnover of birds, the industry must continually breed more, but half of the chicks who hatch are, inevitably, male. They're the wrong sex to lay eggs, and the wrong breed for meat, and so millions of baby birds are killed on their very first day of life. In the UK, they're gassed to death. In Australia and the US, they may instead be fed alive into mincing machines. Being hatched into a 'high-welfare' system won't save them; this same fate awaits male chicks hatched on free-range and organic farms. For more information on 'high-welfare' farming, see page 155.

COWS

Cows possess many of the same emotional qualities as people. Like us, some are playful, cheeky and outgoing, while others are more sensitive, thoughtful or shy. All are capable of happiness, though, and cows literally jump for joy when given reason to. But cows reared for their milk and meat suffer both physically and emotionally.

Like all female mammals, cows must be pregnant to produce milk. On farms, this is usually done via artificial insemination, with one hand in the cow's anus to manipulate her cervix while the other inserts a straw of semen into her vagina. Suddenly, milk doesn't seem quite so natural, does it?

The milk she produces is, of course, intended for her calf but instead of suckling for a year, the young are taken away from their mums within hours of birth to stop them drinking all that valuable milk. Male calves are often deemed worthless and may be shot at birth. Some are reared as veal or trucked straight to the slaughterhouse.[8] Females, who will go on to become 'milkers' themselves, may be moved to hutches where, instead of receiving the comfort, warmth and security that newborns need from their mothers, they are kept confined and alone.

The separation is traumatic for both mother and calf. They call for one another, sometimes for days, with some mothers pacing back and forth, searching for a way to be reunited with their lost young. A cow used by the dairy trade will lose calf after calf as she is repeatedly impregnated, near-continuously milked, and pushed up to and beyond her biological limits. When her milk production declines or she is unable to get pregnant again, she is considered 'spent' and will be sent to slaughter. She could have lived to 20 years old, but will be killed at just five or six, and her body made into low-grade meat products. Even heavily pregnant dairy cows are slaughtered[9] [10] [11] [12] – because of illness or age, or because the farmer did not know they were pregnant[13] – with some calves being born and dying on the slaughterhouse floor.

In some areas of the world, like New Zealand, cows live outdoors all year round because the climate allows it.[14] In other parts of the world, cows farmed for their milk are turned out to graze for around six months of the year, and the rest of the time they stand around in a barn. An increasing number of cows are not allowed outside at all but are instead intensively farmed. After all, why waste valuable time getting cows in from fields when you could just keep them in and bring food to them? This is called 'zero-grazing' and is exactly what it sounds like: the cows never graze. Permanently housing cows inside can lead to two common causes of suffering: mastitis – which is a painful infection of their udders – and lameness, meaning they will struggle to walk, usually due to crippling pain.

Life is no picnic for cows reared for their meat either. Calves may be dehorned, castrated and branded, often all at once. All of these legally permitted mutilations may be performed without anaesthetic[15] and, in most countries, no pain relief is required by law.

Whether they are 'grass-raised' or kept in intensive systems where they never see the outdoors, their lives are over when they reach the required weight. Typically they are just 18 months old;[16] naturally, they could have lived for 20 years or more.

PIGS

Pigs are every bit as intelligent, fun-loving and charismatic as dogs. Yet pigs are reared on intensive farms in a way that would horrify us – and lead to animal cruelty charges – if it were done to our canine friends.

Gestation crates – metal enclosures that confine female pigs throughout each 16-week pregnancy – are banned in the UK, but are still legal in Canada, Australia and most US states.[17] Even in the countries where gestation crates are banned, farrowing crates remain legal. Female pigs may be held in these tiny pens, barely bigger than their own bodies, for several weeks while they complete their pregnancy and give birth. The crates are so small the sows cannot even turn round.

In the wild, pigs would find a private place to build a nest in which to give birth. On farms, all they have are the metal bars that prevent them moving and a concrete or metal floor that can cause painful pressure sores. In desperation, they go through the motions of nest-building, but without any nesting materials available to them; it is, of course, totally futile.[18]

When born, the piglets are able to suckle from their mother but she is separated from them by the bars of the crate and is not able to reach them to nurture or nuzzle them. If they are sick, all she can do is watch them die. She will be kept in this confinement until the young are taken from her, then she will be returned to a pen to be impregnated again. And again, and again, until she is exhausted and her body can no longer endure the strain. Then she will be sent to slaughter as a 'cull sow', and her body turned into low-quality products like pork pies and sausages.

Pigs have been bred to have the largest litters possible (as each additional piglet boosts the profits), but this means many piglets are stillborn, or die soon after birth. They rarely receive veterinary care. Undercover investigators regularly find their tiny bodies abandoned in the aisles of the units or dumped inside bin bags.

In nature, weaning is a gradual process, often taking three to four months. On farms, the separation of mother and piglets after just three or four weeks[19] causes distress to them both. As with cows and their calves, it is quite common for them to call out to one another in the vain hope of being reunited.[20]

Soon after birth, piglets will have their tails cut off, their teeth clipped or ground down and, in many countries, they will also be castrated, all without anaesthetic. The pig industry claims that the first two procedures are necessary to prevent piglets from injuring one another. However, pigs rarely harm one another when living wild. It is a problem related to their overcrowded, stressful living conditions, where boredom is rife.

Piglets may be slaughtered from the age of two weeks to produce 'whole suckling pig', but most are killed when they are around four to six months old. Their mothers are put through between three and five pregnancies before they are also slaughtered, usually at around 18 months to two years old.[21] They could have lived to the age of 20.

All this suffering could be spared if we just choose a meat-style veggie sausage over a meat one.

SHEEP

Sheep are farmed for their meat, milk and wool. They are often misunderstood, and derided as being 'stupid' simply because they flock together for protection, in the same way that some birds and fish do. When they feel safe and secure, sheep will show that they are bright and inquisitive, loving and gentle, and often extremely cheeky. On farms, they're just not given the opportunity to be themselves.

If ewes were able to breed naturally, they would give birth in spring. Now, though, many are forced to give birth in the dead of winter so that the meat is already on the shelves by spring and can be marketed as new season lamb.[22] In Australia, more than 10 million lambs die before weaning with birthing difficulties, exposure to cold weather and starvation cited as leading reasons.[23] It's the same sad story around the world.[24, 25]

Have you ever wondered why ewes on farms all give birth around the same time? It's not a natural cycle. It's done deliberately to ensure lambing takes place at a convenient time for the farmer, and is achieved by implanting hormones under the ewes' skin or inserting hormone sponges into their vaginas to synchronise the flock's fertility.[26]

Insemination may be done artificially, too, with the semen

collected from a ram using an artificial vagina or by an electric probe inserted into the ram's anus.[27] The semen is then either introduced through the cervix while the ewe is strapped to a rack, or introduced surgically through the ewe's abdomen.[28] So far, so unnatural.

Left to nature, ewes would give birth to a single lamb. However, through human manipulation, many sheep are now selectively bred to produce two or even three lambs, which is intended to increase the industry's profitability. Since ewes have just two teats, a third lamb will be given to a different ewe, bottle-fed, or force-fed through a tube into his or her stomach.

Because it is common to see sheep in fields and on hillsides, we think their lives are rather enjoyable. But we tend not to be in those fields when they flood,[29] or when the heat of the summer raises the risk of fly strike,[30] or in the depths of winter when snow makes finding food impossible.[31]

On top of this, sheep suffer a host of health problems and are given an array of drugs to try to prevent or manage unpleasant conditions such as scald, foot rot, scrapie, mastitis, and even blindness. Stand and watch a flock of sheep for a few minutes and you will often see lame animals, painfully limping along, trying to keep up with the rest of the flock. Lameness is endemic but research shows that only a minority of farmers implement the recommended practices to prevent it.[32]

Most lambs are slaughtered when they are between three and five months old, although some are killed as young as six weeks old.[33] They might otherwise have lived for ten years or more. Their mothers will also be killed when age, lameness, udder infections or prolapse mean they are no longer profitable.[34]

FISH

It's not so easy to warm to cold-blooded animals, but research shows that fish are smart enough to use tools, can communicate and have distinct personalities, just like people.

Commercial fishing vessels can capture tens of thousands of fish at a time, with animals becoming exhausted as they desperately try to outswim the net. When pulled to the surface, those at the bottom are crushed by the weight of fish above them. The rapid change in pressure causes their swim bladders to overinflate, and their stomachs and intestines to be pushed out through their mouths and anuses. Their eyes distort, bulge and can be pushed out of their sockets.

The animals are then dropped onto the ship's deck, where those who are still alive will suffocate – a process that can take several minutes. Others, like tuna, are hoisted from the water with a hook, and killed by a spike forced through their brains.

In fish farms, fish are packed into small, often filthy enclosures. Death rates are high – more than 10 million farmed salmon died on Scottish farms in 2019[35] – and an array of chemicals is used to try to prevent even more from succumbing. In this stressful environment, many fish will bite off the fins, tails and eyes of others, a distressing and destructive behaviour seen in other factory-farmed animals.

Despite an ever-increasing number of studies that show aquatic species can feel pain, there are still no welfare laws governing the humane slaughter of fish at sea, and in most countries there are no welfare requirements for slaughter on farms, either. With little or no legal protection, some truly terrible things are done to aquatic species. Lobsters and crabs may be boiled alive, while farmed shrimps are deliberately blinded in a procedure designed to boost their fertility. 'Eyestalk ablation', as the industry calls it, happens in almost every shrimp production facility in the world.[36]

'Going vegan is one of my proudest decisions and has made me feel like I'm really doing my part for animals. I feel healthier and more contented that I'm not contributing to the suffering of animals.'

Alice C., Sussex, UK, Veganuary Class of 2017

SLAUGHTERHOUSES

The lives of most farmed animals are based on deprivation, suffering and loss. For most, there is no 'good life', and nor is there a humane death. In the US, the federal laws that are designed to ensure animals are slaughtered humanely specifically exempt chickens, turkeys, ducks, geese, rabbits and fish, which encompasses the vast majority of animals killed.

In the UK, Australia and elsewhere, campaigners have filmed inside slaughterhouses and revealed that the welfare laws that do exist are often ignored, with animals being kicked, beaten and abused to their deaths. The laws that demand animals be stunned before slaughter are often not properly adhered to, and animals may be partially stunned or not stunned at all, and still go to the knife.

But perhaps the most shocking thing seen in these undercover investigations is the fear that animals display: the sheep running in circles, throwing themselves again and again at the walls, the doors, the gates, anywhere to try to find a way out. Some even leap through the hatch that leads to the slaughter room, and land in the blood pit below their bleeding companions.

These investigations have shown cows being shot up to four times in the head with a captive bolt gun in an attempt to stun them. They lie on the ground, looking up at the slaughterman, blinking and waiting for the next attempt. The investigations show the pain of electrical stunning, which all

24

too often imparts a powerful electric shock instead of rendering the animal unconscious. They've shown pigs convulsing and gasping for air as the cage they are in is lowered into a gas chamber.

In these investigations, we see the pitiless nature of this business: the ewe being stunned while her lamb is still suckling from her; the injured pigs, too lame to walk, kicked and prodded and dragged through the slaughterhouse by their ears; the animals screaming in pain on the floor while a worker stands over them, taunting them. The casual indifference to the fear and suffering of these helpless creatures is demonstrated with every kick, punch and blow inflicted. It's the nature of the business that workers must become desensitised to the animals' fear and pain.

Animals in slaughterhouses are not euthanised like a much-loved dog or cat and there is no humane way to kill an animal who does not want to die, but slaughterhouses are particularly ruthless: the slaughter line has to keep moving, and no matter how hard they might try, no animal escapes.

> *'If slaughterhouses had glass walls,*
> *everyone would be vegetarian.'*
>
> Paul McCartney

BEES

We owe bees a lot. We rely on them – and other insect pollinators – for apples, berries, cucumbers, almonds, beans, broccoli, carrots and many more of the foods that we eat and love.[37] Bees collect pollen and nectar from the flowers of these plants, pollinating as they go. Back at the hive, the nectar's content is reduced by being passed from mouth to mouth until it becomes honey. Bees do all this to create food that will see the hive through winter, not because they are worried about what people are going to have on their toast.

Commercial bee-keepers take the honey and substitute it with a sugar-water solution, which has neither the broad range of nutrients the bees need nor the power to protect their immune systems.[38] This, coupled with exposure to pesticides (including the now-infamous neonicotinoids) and destructive varroa mites, means these insects are facing a rough future.

But that's not all. Some commercial bee-keepers kill and replace the queens to ensure that the queen is always young and fertile. They may even 'cull' whole hives after harvesting the honey as it is cheaper than feeding the bees through the winter months. Of course, they wouldn't need feeding if someone hadn't stolen their honey.

For Animals

THANK YOU

We know that this was a tough section to get through. Reading about what animals have to endure so that people can eat their flesh and eggs and even the animals' own food (milk and honey) is emotionally challenging. No matter how hard it is for us to face it, we have to remember how much harder it is for the animals to live it. And it's not just the animals we've mentioned who suffer. Most ducks, turkeys and geese are reared in factory farm sheds like chickens; rabbits are reared in cages like hens; and goats raised for their meat and milk may be kept inside zero-grazing units and never see the light of day.

It's no surprise that the way we farm and slaughter animals is the main reason people give for trying vegan, but it's not the only reason . . .

FOR THE ENVIRONMENT

A growing number of people are eating plant-based foods to help protect the environment. The connection may not be as immediately obvious as with animals – after all, it's pretty clear that eating animals harms them – but what we choose to eat has a direct and significant impact on climate change, deforestation, pollution, water and land usage, as well as on wild animals.

> 'A vegan diet is probably the single biggest way to reduce your impact on planet Earth, not just greenhouse gases, but global acidification, eutrophication, land use and water use. It is far bigger than cutting down on your flights or buying an electric car . . . Avoiding consumption of animal products delivers far better environmental benefits than trying to purchase sustainable meat and dairy.'[1]

These are the words of Joseph Poore, researcher at Oxford University, who led the most comprehensive study to date into the environmental impacts of many different foods. His own research convinced him to become vegan.

GREENHOUSE GAS EMISSIONS

Every link in the chain that brings meat, milk and eggs from farm to table demands energy: the production of fertiliser that is put on the land to grow feed; powering farm machinery; pumping the water animals need from rivers or deep underground; fuelling live animal transportation in trucks or ships; the constant running of the abattoir's slaughter line; the creation of packaging; and the shipping in refrigerated vehicles of meat products all around the world.

Many people think that food miles are the biggest generator of emissions, and that can incentivise people to buy local, but actually these are just a small percentage of the total, and land use changes and on-farm practices account for much more.[2] Eating vegetables that have been flown in from the other side of the world still accounts for fewer emissions than eating beef from cows reared just down the road.

There is no polite way to say this, but animals also release a lot of methane through their belches and farts. Methane has a warming effect 86 times more potent than carbon dioxide over a 20-year timeframe.[3] Nitrous oxide emissions – from the breakdown of animal waste – are also released in large quantities, and this compound has almost 300 times the warming impact of carbon dioxide.[4]

The Food and Agriculture Organization of the United Nations has found that animal agriculture is responsible for at least 14.5 per cent of all human-caused greenhouse gas emissions,[5] which makes animal products more damaging than the exhaust from every plane, car, truck, train and ship on the planet.[6] It's a sobering thought.

WATER

Although the surface of our planet is predominantly water, only three per cent of it is fresh water, and two-thirds of that is held in frozen glaciers or is otherwise unavailable.[7] Already, 1.2 billion people experience severe water scarcity[8] and – with the world's population predicted to grow to 9.1 billion by 2050 and climate change exacerbating the problem – the strain on this most vital natural, life-preserving resource is only going to increase.[9]

Already, rivers, lakes and aquifers are drying up and more than half of the world's wetlands have disappeared. We would be wise to use water sparingly, and yet global agriculture accounts for 85 per cent of human water consumption.[10] And not all agriculture is equal. The thirstiest of all is animal agriculture.

One study into the water footprints of different foods estimated that vegetables and fruits required 322 and 962 litres per kilogram yield respectively. The water requirement for meat, however, was very much larger: 4,325 litres per kilogram of chicken, 5,988 litres for pork, 8,763 litres for sheep or goat meat and 15,415 per kilogram of beef.[11]

It takes so much more water to produce food for a meat-eater than it does to feed a vegan, and we cannot afford to waste a drop of this precious resource.

POLLUTION

Animal agriculture pollutes our land, waterways and air.

There are billions of farmed animals on this planet, and all of them produce waste. A *lot* of waste. In the days when there was small-scale farming the manure could simply be spread on the land, but we have gone way beyond that recycling of nutrients now. A single cow produces up to 64kg of manure per day[12] and there are one billion cows on the planet.[13] Add to that the billions of other farmed animals – including pigs, sheep, goats, chickens, turkeys, geese, ducks – and it is obvious that the land cannot absorb that much waste. Instead, it is stored in giant, specially built slurry lagoons where, all too often, it leaks out, or overflows and gets into the waterways. Here, it threatens drinking supplies, damages wetlands[14] and fuels 'algal blooms' (the rapid accumulation of algae that wipe out aquatic life).[15] Tens of thousands of miles of rivers in the US, Europe and Asia are polluted with slurry each year,[16] while ocean dead zones are growing in number and size.[17]

To add to the destruction, noxious gases including ammonia escape these lagoons. Ammonia is a major contributor to acid rain, and two-thirds of man-made ammonia is generated by farmed animals.[18] It also harms people. Research has shown that those who work inside large-scale factory farms (known in the US as Concentrated Animal Feeding Operations or CAFOs) are more likely to suffer from asthma and respiratory infections.[19] Worldwide, farm workers continue to die from inhalation of methane emitted from the slurry pits.

Not all the waste is stored in lagoons; some is still sprayed onto fields, but there is just too much of it and when large amounts are sprayed, fine dust particles and ammonia are released into the air and carried into the lungs of local residents. In 2015, Dutch researchers found that people living within a kilometre of 15 or more farms had reduced lung function. One of the main culprits they cited was ammonia.[20]

DEFORESTATION

Feeding a meat-eating population requires much more land than is needed to grow food for a vegan population and, with demand growing, that land must come from somewhere. Inevitably, the farming industry turns its attention to forests and other important habitats, and razes them to the ground to make way for grazing or to grow feed for farmed animals. The largest single cause of deforestation is agriculture.[21]

Approximately 450,000 square kilometres of deforested Amazon in Brazil are now grazed by cows.[22] Once the cows have stripped the area, they are moved to another region where the forest has been deliberately burnt for that purpose, leaving the soya farmers to move into the original space. It would be easy to blame vegetarians and vegans for soya grown on deforested Amazon land but there are two reasons why that would be wrong: first, the forest was destroyed to graze cows with soya being a secondary industry; but also, 80 per cent of that soya is actually grown to feed animals like chickens, pigs and even fish in factory farms around the world, including in the UK.[23] Thanks to global meat consumption, the Amazon is in real trouble with more than half of all tree species there – including Brazil nut, wild cacao and acai – at risk of extinction.[24]

It's not just the Amazon that is being decimated; all forests are under threat from agriculture. Take the great forests of Sumatra and Borneo, for instance. Once full of tigers, elephants, rhinos and orangutans, the habitat has been trashed in just one generation.[25] And for what? In large part, it is for palm plantations – a monoculture, doused with herbicides and pesticides that creates a barren landscape and wipes out wild populations.[26] Most of us know that palm products are found in many of the packaged foods on our supermarket shelves; what is less visible is that palm – like soya – is widely used in animal feed.[27]

Palm oil in plant-based food is a hot topic that is frequently debated on vegan forums. It's your call on how you decide to manage this troublesome ingredient – but you can take comfort in the knowledge that being vegan significantly reduces your unwitting involvement in deforestation practices.

Deforestation is devastating for indigenous communities as well as the animals who rely on the habitat. It is also devastating for our planet in its entirety. Trees play a critical role in absorbing greenhouse gases and when they are logged or burned down to clear land for agriculture, huge quantities of climate-changing gases are released into the atmosphere.[28] The damage does not end when trees are felled and the animals are driven out of their habitats. Forest soils below the canopy are moist but, without trees to protect them from the sun and the wind, they dry out quickly. The soil becomes more fragile, erodes and can wash away during periods of rain. All too often, the once-rich land becomes utterly barren.

WILDLIFE

Humanity has wiped out 60 per cent of bird, mammal, fish and reptile populations since 1970,[29] with many scientists believing we have unleashed the world's sixth mass extinction, and the first to be caused by a species: humans.

Deforestation is one cause of this unprecedented loss of wildlife. Even if we stopped cutting down forests right this moment, we could not be able to stop the decline of animal populations completely. It takes time for a species to die out after trees are felled, so it is predicted that 80-90 per cent of extinctions caused by damage done between 1970 and 2008 are still to come.[30]

Deforestation is just one part of a widespread ecological assault by the agriculture industry. In the UK, populations of farmland birds have fallen 55 per cent in the past 50 years. The government has stated that these declines are 'largely due to the impact of rapid changes in farmland management', including the intensification of farming, increased pesticide and fertiliser use and the removal of hedgerows.[31]

It's the same devastating story across the world. There is an alarming decrease in the number of birds across Europe, with one-third of all species in Germany undergoing a dramatic decline. According to figures released by the German government, species in agricultural areas suffer the worst losses.[32]

Wetland drainage, the conversion of pastureland to cropland (to grow feed for intensively farmed animals) and overgrazing have meant a loss of 70 per cent of the native Canadian prairies, and a 40 per cent decline in their bird populations since the 1970s.[33]

Australia has one of the highest rates of species extinction in the world.[34] In the state of Queensland alone, 90 per cent of woody vegetation clearing is driven by livestock production[35] and this is estimated to kill more than 30 million native mammals, birds and reptiles every year.[36]

A 2019 State of Nature report said: 'Agricultural intensification, driven by UK and European policy, has been identified as the most significant factor driving the decline in species' populations across the UK'.[37]

Of the 8,688 threatened or near-threatened species worldwide, 63 per cent are threatened by agriculture alone, with the cheetah, the African wild dog and the hairy-nosed otter among the most affected.[38] Agriculture and overexploitation (including fishing) were found to be significantly greater threats to biodiversity than climate change.[39]

At the heart of the issue is just how much land is needed to produce animal products. Research suggests that if we all shifted to a plant-based diet, we would reduce global land use by 75 per cent,[40] and that land could go back to nature, and reverse the devastating decline in wildlife and wild spaces.

'We must change our diet. The planet can't support billions of meat-eaters.'

David Attenborough

DEPLETED OCEANS

When we think of modern fishing vessels, we may picture the brightly painted recreational boats we see when we visit the coast. Instead, we should conjure up the image of a vessel the length of Buckingham Palace[41][42] or closer to the size of the Sydney Opera House[43] sweeping the oceans and dragging tonnes of sea creatures into nets that are big enough to enclose 13 jumbo jets.[44]

It's little wonder then that more than 90 per cent of the marine fish populations in the world have been 'fully exploited, overexploited or depleted', according to the United Nations Conference on Trade and Development[45], and whole populations are on the verge of collapse.[46]

This is bad enough, but nets do not discriminate. They drag any species out of the water, whether they are commercially valuable or not. Animals caught unintentionally are known as 'by-catch', and more than 600,000 marine mammals a year, including whales, dolphins and porpoises are caught and drowned.[47] Entire species, including the endangered Maui's dolphin and North Atlantic right whale, are being pushed to the brink of extinction. [48][49]

Sharks,[50] turtles, starfish, sponges and hundreds of thousands of diving seabirds[51] – among them the extraordinary and iconic albatross – are also killed by the nets.

It's not just our taste for wild-caught fish that is driving this destruction. Wild fish are caught and turned into feed for farmed animals, including chickens and farmed fish. Our consumption of all kinds of animal products is devastating the oceans.

In recent years, another threat to the health of our oceans has become apparent – plastic. While we cut our use of plastic straws and disposable coffee cups, what we are not told is that dumped and lost fishing gear from commercial enterprises is by far the biggest oceanic plastic polluter.[52]

SUSTAINABILITY
AND WORLD HUNGER

Until we work out how to colonise Mars, we have just the
one planet to live on, and this little orb must sustain billions
of people and millions of other species, too. There are finite
resources and we need to share them and take care of them.
Currently, our desire for meat means that not everyone can
be fed.

The world already produces enough food to feed every
person on the planet and 2.5 billion more,[1] yet one in nine
people still do not get enough food to be healthy.[2] One key
issue is that, instead of feeding people, we feed the grain to
farmed animals who are inefficient converters of feed
to meat. In simple terms, we get back fewer calories than
we feed them. Pigs, for example, require 8.4kg of feed to
produce 1kg of meat, while chickens require 3.4kg of feed
to produce 1kg.[3] For every 100 calories of grain we feed to
farmed animals, we get back only about 40 new calories of
milk, 22 calories of eggs, 12 of chicken, 10 of pork or three

of beef.[4] It's incredibly wasteful and no way to feed a growing population

The Food and Agriculture Organization of the United Nations puts it this way: 'When livestock are raised in intensive systems, they convert carbohydrate and protein that might otherwise be eaten directly by humans and use them to produce a smaller quantity of energy and protein.'[5] No wonder UK thinktank Chatham House describes feeding cereals to animals as 'staggeringly inefficient'.[6]

If we were to start from scratch, get our greatest minds round a boardroom table and ask them to devise the best way to use the world's resources and efficiently feed the human population, this plan would be laughed out of the room.

Of course, there are other reasons for hunger – including war, poverty and natural disasters – but there is already enough food for all of us so long as we stop feeding it to farmed animals.

FOR PERSONAL HEALTH

'I'd say that within about a week I felt like a different
person. I've always had different health problems. I
used to have stomach problems. I got a lot of ulcers.
I got a lot of acid problems. They cleared up. My
mental health was definitely helped. Absolutely give it
a go. Why not? It's only a month!'

Carl Donnelly, comedian,
UK and Veganuary Ambassador

WHAT VEGANUARY PARTICIPANTS
FOUND AFTER 31 DAYS

Each year, people who take part in Veganuary are asked how
they found their month of plant-based eating and what physical changes they experienced during that time. Among the
most common responses are: my skin cleared up; my

digestion is a whole lot better; my sinuses are clearer; my nails are stronger; I have more energy.

Others tell us that they sleep better, have stopped snoring and experience increased libido. For some women, their periods are easier, while others have reported an improvement in their menopause symptoms. One person wrote: 'I didn't realise how "sick" my body felt 'til I realised what "healthy" feels like.'

We regularly hear that eczema, psoriasis and acne improve or clear up, and those who suffer irritable bowel syndrome (IBS) often report that the symptoms decrease in severity or disappear altogether. One participant said her chronic fatigue symptoms improved, another that her chronic muscle pain had disappeared. Several people report that their arthritis symptoms eased, with one woman saying, 'My joint pain has gone for the first time in my life.'

Sporty people often find that being vegan helps them recover from training quicker, and that allows them to train even harder and achieve more impressive results. Others are just amazed that they are able to effectively build muscle and endurance on a plant-based diet.

'As a boxer my weight is constantly watched and has to be managed. Simply from changing to a vegan diet (not "dieting"), I lost weight without trying to and I also have noticed I am leaner and carry less body fat now compared to before. My coach noticed a difference in my training, particularly in terms of endurance. I could work harder for longer without tiring as much as I used to, like I was running off a better fuel source. I used to think I wouldn't be able to get enough protein to fuel my training and recovery if I went vegan, but that has not been the case at all.'

Shereen H., Sheffield, UK, Class of 2020

What is really interesting is the number of people who report better mental clarity, increased concentration and a levelling out of moods. Some participants tell us that their depression symptoms were relieved. For lots of people, eating animal-free foods brings an unexpected contentment, a feeling of inner peace, brought on by eating a diet more in line with their beliefs and principles.

We can't promise everyone that their niggling conditions and chronic illnesses will disappear after 31 days of plant-based eating, but for lots of people, a month without eating animal products brings a stark, often unexpected, improvement.

> *'Most deaths in the United States are*
> *preventable, and they are related to what*
> *we eat.'*
>
> Dr Michael Greger, author of *How Not to Die*

HEART DISEASE

Heart disease is the number one cause of death worldwide,[1] and lifestyle factors play a big part. We know, of course, that smoking is bad, that exercise is good and that we should limit alcohol intake and stress. But what about diet?

Research shows that putting plants at the centre of our meals can reduce many of the risk factors for heart disease, including high cholesterol levels, high blood pressure, being overweight and developing type 2 diabetes.

- The first risk factor is cholesterol. Animal products contain it whereas plant products don't.[2] And consuming saturated fat – the kind found in processed and fatty meats, hard cheeses, whole milk, cream and butter[3] causes the liver to produce more cholesterol,[4] which contributes to the formation of plaques. These clog up our arteries, making a heart attack or stroke more likely.

- High blood pressure is another risk factor for heart disease. This is a condition that often cannot be felt, which means there are no warning signs that you may be at risk. Lifestyle factors including diet and exercise are all-important, and once again vegans have been found to have a lower risk.[5]

• A third risk factor is obesity. More than 42 per cent of adult Americans,[6] 31 per cent of adult Australians[7] and more than 28 per cent of adults in England are obese.[8] It's a serious, life-limiting and life-threatening condition, which makes heart disease and stroke more likely. Studies have regularly shown that vegetarians are slimmer, and vegans appear to have the lowest Body Mass Index of all.[9]

Information on type 2 diabetes – the fourth risk factor in developing heart disease and a serious condition in its own right – can be found in the next section.

Studies consistently show that a balanced plant-based diet is a heart-healthy diet. A meta-analysis of research conducted between 1960 and 2018 examined 40 studies featuring 12,619 vegans and 179,630 omnivores. It found that vegans had a lower BMI, smaller waist circumference, lower blood pressure and lower LDL ('bad') cholesterol.[10]

It's never too early to start eating better for your heart, but it is also never too late. Those who have already developed a heart condition may see significant improvements from switching to a plant-based diet.[11]

'As a diabetic it's really important I keep good control of my blood sugar and also try to limit the effects of this illness such as increased risk of heart and vascular disease. Controlling my cholesterol is the best thing I can do along with trying to control my weight. I had my cholesterol tested at the end of 2019, before I started Veganuary, then again about 4 months later – I was amazed to see my reading come down a whole point, and my diabetic specialist team were delighted to see such a change in a short space of time. This is attributed to there being no animal saturated fat in my diet furring up my arteries. Changing to this way of life may have actually helped me live longer and healthier.'

Emma G. Fife, UK, Class of 2020

TYPE 2 DIABETES

Unlike type 1 diabetes, type 2 is largely lifestyle-related, with obesity being the greatest risk factor.[12]

In his book *How Not to Die*, Dr Michael Greger describes how the condition comes about:

The number of fat cells in your body doesn't change much in adulthood, no matter how much weight you gain or lose. They just swell up with fat as the body gains weight, so when your belly gets bigger, you're not necessarily creating new fat cells; rather you're just cramming more fat into the existing ones. In overweight and obese people, these cells can get so bloated that they actually spill fat back into the bloodstream.[13]

Type 2 diabetes is a very serious condition. Complications arising from it include heart disease and stroke, nerve damage, kidney disease, sexual dysfunction, sight loss and blindness, leg ulcers and peripheral vascular disease that can lead to foot or limb amputation. These serious complications are horribly common. Diabetes is the leading cause of blindness in working age Australians,[14] while in England, the number of diabetes-related amputations has reached an all-time high of 176 per week.[15]

Type 2 diabetes is a potentially devastating condition and yet in most people it can be prevented or managed through simple lifestyle changes, and it can even be reversed in those who have already developed it. Researchers studying diet and diabetes concluded: 'The benefits of all types of vegetarian diets in the prevention and treatment of diabetes have been well established . . . However, there is evidence that a vegan diet has the most benefits for reducing the fasting plasma glucose levels of persons with diabetes and other complications, such as CVD [cardiovascular disease] risk.'[16]

The interesting thing is that it isn't just about weight. Even at the same weight as meat-eaters, vegans appear to have less risk of diabetes.[17] This may be down to the difference in fats consumed, but whatever the cause, cutting out animal products and eating plant-based foods reduces the risk of developing this dreadful condition.

> 'Plant-based foods, particularly fruit and vegetables, nuts, pulses and seeds, have been shown to help in the treatment of many chronic diseases and are often associated with lower rates of type 2 diabetes, less hypertension, lower cholesterol levels and reduced cancer rates.'[18]
>
> *Diabetes UK*

CANCERS

In 2015, World Health Organization scientists felt they had amassed enough evidence from decades of work to state categorically that all processed meat causes cancer, while red meat is a 'probable' cause.[19] This means that bacon, sausages, hot dogs, ham, salami and pepperoni are now officially classified as carcinogens, just as tobacco is.[20] They warned that eating 50g of processed red meat a day – that's less than two slices of bacon – raises the risk of colon cancer by 18 per cent.[21] Immediately after the announcement, sales of bacon and sausages fell sharply.[22]

It's not just the meat itself but how it's cooked that can cause trouble. Whenever meat – including beef, chicken and fish – is cooked at high temperatures, chemicals called heterocyclic amines (HCAs) form, and these are also carcinogenic.[23] The longer meat is cooked, the more HCAs form, and this may explain why eating well-done meat is associated with increased risk of colorectal, pancreatic and prostate cancer.[24] Of course, *not* cooking meat thoroughly is connected to a greater risk of food-borne infections and food poisoning[25] so there is risk in meat-eating either way.

Recent scientific studies have suggested that dairy products may be linked to an increased risk for breast[26] and prostate cancer.[27] This may be down to dairy consumption boosting the hormone IGF-1 (insulin-like growth factor 1) in the bloodstream or it may be the amount of calcium ingested, but there are other possible mechanisms being studied and more work is needed to show a conclusive link.

'It's the position of the Academy of Nutrition and Dietetics that appropriately planned vegetarian, including vegan, diets are healthful, nutritionally adequate and may provide health benefits for the prevention and treatment of certain diseases. Vegetarians and vegans are at reduced risk of certain health conditions, including ischemic heart disease, type 2 diabetes, hypertension, certain types of cancer, and obesity.'[28]

The Academy of Nutrition and Dietetics

FOR GLOBAL HEALTH

DISEASES FROM FARMED ANIMALS

Damaging as animal products can be to our individual health, this is nothing compared with what animal agriculture can do to human health at a global level. Did you know that many of the common diseases that make us sick originated in animals we farmed? It is thought that measles originally came from the rinderpest virus in cows, whooping cough from pigs, leprosy from water buffalo, the common cold from horses and influenza from poultry.[1] The consumption of animals also allowed other viruses to transmit to people including HIV, SARS, MERS and, of course, COVID-19. In fact, three quarters of all emerging infectious diseases in people come from animals.[2]

The most serious strain of bird flu is H5N1, which has a mortality rate in people of 60 per cent.[3] Thankfully, it doesn't pass easily from person to person which is why most of us know little about it. But pandemic experts have long kept an eye on factory farms, especially pig and chicken farms, where high densities of animals with already compromised immune systems[4] provide the ideal environment for new influenza strains to evolve.[5]

Farming and eating animals has been harming us for centuries, and unless we learn some lessons, our meat habit will continue to wreak havoc on public health.

ANTIBIOTICS

Intensive farming is a practice that stresses animals and weakens their immune systems while simultaneously exposing them to squalor. No surprise, then, that disease on such farms is rife. But instead of providing better conditions, the industry doses the animals with antibiotics.

Antibiotics are the wonder drugs that changed modern medicine and have saved countless human lives since their discovery less than one hundred years ago. But we've become complacent. We take them when we don't need them, or don't finish the prescribed course. And globally we add them to the feed of farmed animals, whether they need them or not, often just because of their growth-promoting qualities. By overusing them like this, we have allowed resistant strains of superbugs to emerge.

Dame Sally Davies, now the UK Special Envoy on Microbial Resistance, has warned of an 'apocalyptic scenario'[6] where diseases become resistant to all types of antibiotics. Dr Margaret Chan, former Director-General of the World Health Organization (WHO), has said 'we face a post-antibiotic era, in which many common infections will no longer have a cure and, once again, kill unabated'.[7] The British government has spoken about 'ten million deaths per year' if something is not done.[8]

WHO has warned of a growing number of infections that are becoming harder to treat, among them pneumonia, tuberculosis, gonorrhoea and salmonellosis. It describes antibiotic resistance as 'one of the biggest threats to global health, food security, and development today.'[9]

Meat production accounts for around 73 per cent of global antibiotic use.[10] Princeton University researchers describe a 'smorgasbord of antibiotic consumption for livestock that has tripled the occurrence of antibiotic resistance in disease-causing bacteria.'[11]

FOR FAITH

There is no religion on Earth that says its followers must be vegan but then none say you shouldn't be vegan either. All major faiths deal with the bigger questions of life, including those about the nature of the world, our role in it and our individual responsibilities and morality. Each has a set of ethical beliefs and guides its followers how to lead a 'good' life. It is not surprising then that those who ask themselves these kinds of questions are increasingly coming to the conclusion that farming and eating animals may not fit with their own ethical and compassionate beliefs.

For some, it is hard to square the intrinsic suffering inside factory farms and slaughterhouses with their own commitment to a peaceable life. For others, climate change – and its disproportionate impact on the world's poorest – inspires them to make changes in their own lives so that they can live more equitably. And for others, the impact of animal agriculture on the world's wild places – on nature or the Creation, perhaps – lead them to question whether we might have taken a wrong path.

There are now vegan Christian, Jewish, Muslim, Buddhist, Sikh and Hindu groups and organisations, and each sets out their own reasons for pursuing and promoting a plant-based path. Those with an interest in finding out more about how veganism is an expression of their own religious teachings can follow or join these groups.

And, of course, there are many more people who feel a spiritual connection that does not align with any one religion but is nonetheless a guiding principle in their lives. They may try to live compassionately and peacefully, tread lightly on the Earth, and prioritise kindness and love. It is easy to see why veganism can play such a significant part in people's spiritual lives.

Veganism isn't a religion, but it fits within many ideologies, and followers of all faiths find that veganism is a way to express their own beliefs and values through their daily actions.

'It is the one decision that has unified the spiritual, physical, mental and emotional side of my humanity. I feel in harmony with animals, and feel that my veganism affirms my desire and commitment to do no harm to animals and the environment. I'm finally living long-held values and morals.'

Jennie R., California, USA

FOR THE ADVENTURE

There are lots of great reasons to try vegan for 31 days. Most people will say they are doing it for the animals, for the environment or for their own health. But some people do it just because. For them it is a challenge, to see what it would be like, to see if they can do it and to see how their life might change.

For everyone, though, there is a period of adjustment – of learning, finding new foods and recipes and sometimes discovering new ways of cooking. Almost everyone reports that, where they had expected to feel more limited in their food choices, instead a whole new world of amazing ingredients opens up before them.

Research shows that most of us cook just nine different meals on a repetitive loop, even though we may own several recipe-packed cookbooks.[1] We get stuck in a rut, and as a result we lose all passion for our food.

'There is so much variety out there, and I think my taste buds have changed since I eat so much more fresh wholefoods – food just tastes that much better.'
Emily J., London, UK, Veganuary Class of 2017

It's easily done but people who take part in Veganuary often say that the culinary shake-up means they are trying foods they have never tried before. They are making new meals and rediscovering their love of great food. But they also find that shops are full of vegan convenience foods, so on the days when they feel like pie and mash or vegan chicken and chips, that's exactly what they can have.

The fact that 98 per cent of people who take part in Veganuary would recommend it to others shows just how much fun those 31 days can be. The most common response to the question: *What advice would you give to someone thinking about trying vegan for 31 days?* is: *Do it. There is nothing to lose and so much to gain.*

'I started this for health reasons and was fully intending to "suffer" my way through January eating plant-based and then celebrate the 1st of Feb with an omni feast. The thing is I've found that my health has improved massively and I've been wondering why the hell I would go back to eating animal products when I just don't need to.'

Samantha H. Class of 2021

SO, WHAT WILL I ACHIEVE?

'It's like having an epiphany and, to begin with, you want to shout what you have learned from the rooftops. I have made some great friends online, I have made some great friends in the "free-from" aisle in my local supermarket! I'm 28 pounds lighter and now run three times a week as part of my vegan running club. To say it has improved several aspects of my life for the better would be an understatement!'

Laura-Jayne W., Shropshire, UK,
Veganuary Class of 2017

Everyone who tries vegan for 31 days gets something different out of it. For some, their health improves radically. The niggles, illnesses and conditions they once experienced clear up, and they are left with a new vigour, a newfound confidence and a much brighter future. Amateur and professional athletes report training benefits and say they wish they had done it sooner.

Lots of people lose weight, which is great if they wanted to. Those whose weight is on the low side, too, are often pleased to see they can make these dietary changes without losing additional weight just by making informed food choices.

But not everyone will notice an instantaneous, miraculous change. For some people, the fact that *nothing* changes is what is so great – they can still cook tasty food, feel the same as they did before and can still eat out with friends in local restaurants. They're just doing it all plant-based.

Those who have struggled with the realities of animal farming – perhaps they have seen reports in newspapers or online about the treatment of animals – say they feel that a weight has been lifted from them. They never wanted to be part of the cruelty, but they did not know how to separate themselves from it. For them, a clearer conscience changes their whole outlook on life. Bringing practice in line with principles is also a wonderful outcome for those concerned about our planet, its wild spaces and its inhabitants.

One interesting consequence is that some people say they feel more connection with nature. Understanding the impact of our food choices inevitably rings some alarm bells, but it also makes us more aware of how beautiful and fragile this planet is. Lots of people say they enjoy being out in nature more, and they feel a greater sense of connection, empathy and even compassion, which spills into every part of their lives.

There are so many possible outcomes and we can't say for sure how being vegan will change *your* life. There is only one way to find that out.

HOW TO GO VEGAN

• • •

This is the big question – how exactly do we make this change in our lives? Since most of us were brought up eating meat, milk and eggs, switching to a new way of eating is a big deal and it's natural to think about – and worry about – what we'll miss when leaving these products behind. But going vegan doesn't have to feel like a huge sacrifice. In fact, it really should not feel anything like that at all!

Some people – but not all – find that it's easier to switch one product at a time, so it doesn't seem like an overwhelming overhaul of their diet. They may try various brands of meat-free sausages or burgers to start with, then decide to stick to one that they like best. They may find that the faux fish fingers taste just like real fish, and start to include these in their diet before switching to dairy-free yoghurts and milks. Others leap right in, clear their fridge of all things animal-based and go vegan overnight. And, of course, many find that trialling veganism for one month – with plenty of support from Veganuary but without any notion of a long-term plant-based commitment – allows people to embrace it, get used to it and treat it as an adventure. Whatever is right for you is the right way. And whether you're a toe-dipper or a cannon-baller into the world of veganism, you can get the tastes, textures and flavours you love without the animal suffering, cholesterol and poor environmental record. You just need to know where to look!

Like all new habits and lifestyles, there will be a period of adjustment while you learn which foods are vegan and where to find them, but it really won't take long before you're veganing like a pro. There is not space in this book to share with you all the great brands and products you can find in your local shops, but what we can do is to point you in the right direction and then it's over to you to do a little research of your own.

Before we get started, a brief word of advice about putting pressure on yourself: please don't. If you're keen to try veganism but find you fall off the wagon, don't assume that veganism is not for you. You just made a mistake. That's OK, we're all human, and we've all done it. Just start again. Every day you eat plant-based is a wonderful thing, so don't worry too much about the odd hiccup.

WHAT TO DO FIRST

The last thing you want to do is wake up on 1 January – or whatever date you've chosen to start your vegan odyssey – and find there's nothing for breakfast but dry bread and black tea. With such a desperate start to the day, you'll come to the rapid conclusion that veganism sucks, and we'd be surprised if you were still vegan at lunchtime. With just a little planning, though, you'll find that a vegan breakfast can be surprisingly similar to a non-vegan one. So before you begin, ask yourself this: *What do I normally eat for breakfast?*

If cereal is your thing, you'll find that lots of cereals are vegan, but you will need to watch out for honey and switch to a plant-based milk. There are so many non-dairy milks available now – including soya, oat, rice, hemp, coconut, almond and cashew – and different tastes suit different people. It's true that none of them taste exactly like cows' milk because they're not the same thing, and we only drink cows' milk in any case because that's what we're used to. Experiment with different varieties until you find the ones you like best. It may be that almond is perfect for your coffee but you prefer oat on your cereal. Mix it up, and see what works for you.

If you like toast, you'll find most breads are vegan and dairy-free spreads are available in every mainstream shop as well as in many health food shops. Jam, marmalade, peanut butter and yeast extracts like Marmite are all vegan anyway, so your toast need never be naked.

You'll find dairy-free yoghurts are readily available, and most people can't tell them apart from the dairy versions. Top them off with nuts, seeds and fruit. Fruit is good – eat lots! And why not allow your newly found adventurous spirit to lead you to the fruits you've never picked up in the super-market before? You know the ones – those weirdly shaped, hairy, spiky, slightly scary ones? Some are an acquired taste but most taste beautiful.

If you're a Big Breakfast Person, that's good, too. Hash browns and baked beans are fine. Add in some vegan sausages and bacon, and top up with tomatoes and mushrooms or avocado. You can even make scrambled tofu if you'd like, and it is surprisingly similar to scrambled egg. And don't worry – ketchup is vegan, too, as are coffee, tea and fruit juices.

So, you've had a three-course breakfast and your day is off to a flying start. But unless you want to eat the same foods for *every* breakfast, lunch and dinner, you'll need to branch out. Our advice in those first few days is not to get too radical. If you normally eat soup for lunch, find a vegan soup to enjoy. If you like a casserole for your dinner, make a vegan version. There will be plenty of time to don an apron and create avocado gazpacho with Egyptian dukkah dust, but for now there's nothing wrong with sticking to what you know.

If you're not sure whether a product you normally buy is vegan, check out the label-reading section in this book. You can also search online, or ask within the Veganuary Facebook group. Whatever you do, please don't give up just because you don't know whether your favourite sandwich pickle is vegan. (By the way, it probably is.)

THE CHEESE ADDICTION

Before we get into the nuts and seeds of veganising your life, we want to address the problem of cheese. Often when someone is struggling to become vegan, cheese is the thing that holds them back. It's almost as if that stuff is addictive! In fact, researchers have found that the casein in cheese can trigger the brain's opioid receptors, which produces a feeling of euphoria.[1] This may explain, in part, why cheese often seems to be the thing that new vegans miss the most.

But cheese is not addictive in the same way drugs are addictive. Anyone can give it up, although we know it can take some mighty willpower, at least to begin with.

To make it that bit easier, we'd suggest you avoid the cheese aisle in your local supermarket when you first become vegan – after all, why risk the temptation? But you'll be pleased to know that dairy-free cheeses have come a very long way in the past few years. Every major supermarket carries several varieties and there are dozens, perhaps hundreds, more available online. Of course, they won't taste exactly like dairy cheese because they're not dairy cheese – and no two dairy cheeses taste the same anyway. But some vegan cheeses taste *really* good, so pile up the crackers and pickles and have your very own vegan cheese-taster session to find out which are the ones for you.

If you're cooking with it, be aware that some vegan cheeses melt and some don't. If you're struggling to find the perfect topping for your pizza, go along to any of the mainstream pizza restaurants in the UK where excellent, melting, dairy-free cheese can be added to your meal.

If you steer clear of dairy cheese for 31 days, something unexpected might well happen to you. Lots of vegans report that, where once they would push their noses up against the cheese counter, trying to inhale it even if they'd decided against eating it, very quickly after going vegan the smell of cheese becomes less appealing. Unpleasant, even. Rancid and sweaty-sock-ish. Our taste buds also change very quickly, and once the cheese habit is broken, you may find that you're completely turned off by the very thing that you once missed so much.

But if after everything you find that you absolutely cannot go without dairy cheese, just be vegan apart from the cheese. An all-or-nothing approach is not helpful here, and an almost-vegan is a whole lot better for animals and the planet than a not-vegan-at-all. So, eat your vegan meals, adding cheese where you want it, but do keep trying the different dairy-free cheeses, too. One day, it might all just click.

VEGAN AT HOME

SURPRISINGLY VEGAN FOODS

The biggest concern for people contemplating a vegan diet is almost always: *What will I eat?* There is a notion that there are specialist vegan products that taste like cardboard and are only found on dusty shelves in out-of-the-way shops, and that all the old favourites must be relinquished. This is so very far from the truth.

Take a look inside any meat-eater's kitchen and you'll find a great number of everyday store-cupboard products that are already vegan. They weren't designed for vegans, but they contain no animal products at all, and include items we eat regularly and couldn't imagine life without. Peanut butter, yeast extracts, jams and marmalades, baked beans, dried pasta, rice, almost all bread, many types of gravy granules, vegetable stock cubes, chopped tomatoes, oven chips and hash browns, coconut milk, lots of curry pastes, many breakfast cereals, herbs, spices, pickles, tomato ketchup and HP sauce, mustard and soy sauce, olive oil and vegetable oils, fruit juice, tea and coffee, lots of cookies, crackers, crispbreads and crisps, and of course fruit and vegetables – fresh, dried, tinned and frozen. All vegan.

That's a pretty good start, isn't it?

Having so many everyday products already free from animal parts means that we can make small, almost unnoticeable changes to our existing diet that will transform it from an omnivorous one to a vegan one. We can ease ourselves into veganism with beans on toast (we need only change the butter) or sausages and mash (just choose veggie sausages and vegetable gravy), and it won't seem like the world has shifted beneath our feet. The meal is essentially the same; it just requires a different brand of the same product.

And there are a lot of vegan products out there – from croissants and cookies to pretzels and pies. Check out veganuary.com and look elsewhere online for 'accidentally vegan products' and you'll see just how many there are. If you're craving something and don't know where to look, ask the Veganuary Facebook group – if anyone knows, you'll find the answer there! Think of it as the oracle for all things vegan.

Quite often, the brand you've been buying all along was vegan anyway. You just didn't know it.

Do bear in mind that you may need to alter your shopping habits slightly and you'll soon learn that it's better to be prepared. In some parts of the world, you'd be unlikely to track down vegan cheese at the neighbourhood convenience store and you may need to travel to a supermarket further afield, rely on a health food store with limited opening hours or search for what you want online. You might sacrifice some convenience, but you will gain some awesome organisational skills.

READING LABELS

We won't lie to you. In the first fortnight of being vegan, you are going to read a LOT of food labels and your weekly shopping run is likely to take just that little bit longer. When you start to look at ingredients, you may be shocked to find you have no idea what half of them are, or why you are eating them. *What on Earth is 'casein' and what's it doing in my cracker? And what do you mean I've been eating crushed beetles?*

Since it's better to know what we're putting into our bodies than to go on in ignorance, reading labels at this stage is a good thing, and it won't be forever. Very soon you'll be fluent in this new language, and will just pick up one brand over another without having to check each time. You'll know that D2 is vegan but D3 may not be. You'll know that whey is from milk, and aspic can be made from clarified meat. You'll even know what isinglass is. Just imagine how many people you will wow at dinner parties. Here is our three-step process to get you started when you pick up a package off the shelf:

1. Does it say 'Vegan' on the packaging? Yes? Read no further.

2. Does it say 'Vegetarian' on the package? Yes? That's a good start, but let's examine it more closely. In the UK, across Europe and in the US, Canada and Australia, ingredients that are likely to cause allergies must be declared on the package. These major allergens include milk, egg and fish ingredients. This means if it says it's vegetarian and these allergens are *not* listed, then (providing it doesn't contain any E numbers, which may require further inspection – see below) there is just one more check to make. Is there honey in it? No? Great! It's vegan.

3. Not all companies label things as well as they might. In this case, you will need your forensic head on, and to look at those ingredients separately. At this point, it is common to wonder how such a small package can contain so many ingredients. It can be quite a revelation that the natural, healthy diet we thought we had contains all manner of items we can't identify.

Here are some hidden demons to look out for:

- **Albumen/albumin** – from eggs, and may be used in baked goods

- **Aspic** – an industry alternative to gelatine, and usually made from meat or fish

- **Carmine/cochineal/E120** – the red pigment of crushed female cochineal beetles, used as a food colouring in cakes and sweets

- **Casein** – a protein from milk, may be found in soups, chocolate and baked goods

- **E numbers** – in Europe, E numbers are a feature of many ingredient lists and some of them are animal derived. You can find a list of non-vegan E numbers online, so you know what to look out for

- **Gelatine** – obtained by boiling the skin, tendons, ligaments and bones of cows or pigs, and found in jelly, chewy sweets, cakes and in the capsules of some vitamins

- **Honey** – food for bees, made by bees. Often found in breakfast cereals and cereal bars

- **Isinglass** – derived from the swim bladders of fish, and used in the clarification of some wines and beers. (You won't find this ingredient on a label, though, as strictly speaking it is not an ingredient but a product used in the process. Visit www.barnivore.com for a list of vegan wine, beer and spirits)

- **Lactose** – a sugar from milk, can be found in baked goods

- **Lard** – white pork fat that has been rendered and clarified

- **Propolis** – used by bees in the construction of their hives. May be found in foods claiming specific health benefits

- **Shellac** – the resin secreted by female lac insects, and used as a food glaze

- **Vitamin D3** – it's possible to get vegan vitamin D3, but often it comes from the liver of fish. If the pack says 'vegetarian', you'll know which one you have

- **Whey** – the liquid remaining after milk has been curdled and strained, often found in baked products

4. If you're not a fan of reading labels (believe us, some people are!) or are short on time, you can use an app such as Vegan Scan to check products – set your dietary requirement and get scanning to find out what is safe. Not every product is in the database (that would be a tall order), but more are being added every day.

5. If, after all this, you're really not sure if the product you want to buy is vegan, go online. There are thousands of vegans on social media – including in the Veganuary Facebook group – who will know the answer immediately. Not only will they be able to tell you whether your product is vegan, they will be able to suggest a heap of similar products, too. So, when we say that, far from restricting options, becoming vegan opens up a whole new world of food, we're not kidding.

6. If all else fails, contact the manufacturer. If your favourite brand isn't vegan, contact them anyway and ask why not. Ingredients change all the time, and if a company realises it will sell more by substituting an animal ingredient for a vegan version, it will listen. It may take some time, but it will definitely listen.

Here are three more tips to help you on your way.

1. Don't believe that 'dairy-free' or 'lactose-free' means vegan. Sometimes it does; sometimes it doesn't. It's best to check to see what other ingredients are in there.

2. Lactic acid is vegan. Lactose is not. It's a bit confusing but it's great news for fans of pickles.

3. This may seem confusing, but if a package says 'may contain traces of milk and eggs', it could still be vegan. In some countries, it's mandatory to give this warning if the product has been made in a factory where non-vegan items have been handled but it doesn't mean the product itself isn't vegan. It may help to think of it like this – imagine a friend is making you a vegan sandwich in their kitchen. Just because they've previously prepared non-vegan food in that kitchen, doesn't make the sandwich any less vegan. Be sure to check the ingredient and the allergen lists to see what is actually *in* the product – unless you have an allergy or intolerance, you can disregard these 'cross-contamination' warnings.

VEGAN INGREDIENT ESSENTIALS

While having a kitchen full of versatile and tasty ingredients will be your first step towards making fantastic vegan food, don't feel that you need to rush out in search of white truffle oil this instant. You already have many of the basics in your kitchen, so use this section as a guide to help grow your vegan larder over time.

PROTEIN SOURCES

- **Tofu:** Choose firmer varieties for cooking or silken for sauces and desserts. Plain tofu will soak up flavours and there are many varieties that are already flavoured or marinated

- **Seitan:** A high-protein meat replacement made from wheat gluten, which has a great 'meaty' texture

- **Tempeh:** Similar to tofu in that it's made from fermented soya beans, but is firmer and with a stronger flavour. Try marinating it

- **Peas:** Garden peas or petit pois, frozen or tinned

- **Beans:** Choose from a wide variety, including kidney, cannellini, pinto, black, lima and chickpeas (garbanzo). There are ready-to-eat tinned beans and dried versions that you will need to soak before cooking

- **Lentils:** Puy, red, brown or green. Buy them dried or in pre-packed form, and use them in sauces, stews, curries, bolognese, shepherd's pie, lasagne and whatever else you like

- **Seeds:** Sunflower, pumpkin, sesame, chia, flax. Seeds are packed full of good stuff! Great on cereals, in stir-fries, salads, stews – in fact pretty much anywhere

- **Nuts:** Almonds, cashews, walnuts, Brazils, pine nuts, pistachios, peanuts

- **Nut butters:** You probably already have peanut butter, but did you know you can get others? Almond, cashew and hazelnut are all really tasty

DAIRY REPLACEMENTS

- **Vegetable spread:** Look for the range of dairy-free butters in supermarkets and health food shops. Be aware of buttermilk in otherwise 'plant-based' butters – that's not vegan

- **Dairy-free cheese:** There are many brands and flavours available to try, including hard cheeses, grated and cream cheeses. Some are based on coconut, others on soya or cashews

- **Plant milks:** Try soya, oat, almond, rice, hemp, coconut, cashew and various flavoured milks

- **Yoghurts:** Some are made from soya, others from coconut or oats, and they come in a wide range of flavours. There are Greek-style vegan yoghurts, too

- **Ice cream:** There are ever-growing ranges of vegan ice creams, cones and choc ices in many different flavours. And the big ice cream brands you already know and love are getting in on the act too!

- **Cream:** There are vegan single creams for pouring on desserts or using in soups, whipping cream for cakes and squirty cream in a can for anything you like!

GRAINS

- **Rice:** Choose from brown, white, basmati, jasmine or wild

- **Quinoa:** A high-protein grain that can be used like rice

- **Couscous:** Made from wheat, and available in white, wholewheat and flavoured varieties. Ready in minutes and delicious hot or cold

- **Pasta:** Avoid egg pasta and any coloured with squid ink. Otherwise, all shapes and sizes are good

- **Polenta:** Cornmeal that can be made into porridge/oatmeal, turned into a traditional Mediterranean bake or eaten as a great alternative to mashed potato

- **Oats and millet:** Excellent choices for a hearty breakfast

BAKING

- **Egg replacer:** There are several brands available online and in health food shops; just follow the instructions

- **Flaxseeds:** Can also be used as an egg replacer. One tablespoon of ground flaxseeds with three tablespoons of warm water replaces one egg in cake and pancake recipes

- **Chia seeds:** Another egg replacer. One tablespoon of seeds with two tablespoons of water replaces one egg

- **Coconut oil:** Good for replacing butter but will leave a gentle coconutty flavour so be careful what you use it in

- **Agave nectar:** Great instead of honey

- **Maple syrup:** Another honey replacement

- **Blackstrap molasses / black treacle:** Great binding agents for home-made flapjacks, granola and power bars and a good source of iron and calcium

- **Pastry:** Some of the leading ready-made puff and shortcrust pastry brands are vegan if you don't fancy making your own

CONDIMENTS AND SAUCES

- **Miso:** A traditional Japanese seasoning. Eat as a soup or use as a flavouring

- **Tamari and soy sauce:** Tamari is a thicker, less salty, fermented sauce that contains less wheat than soy sauce

- **Table sauces:** Including barbecue, Thai sweet chilli, ketchup, HP, mint and apple sauces, chutneys and mustards – many everyday brands are vegan

HEALTHY SNACKS

- **Dried fruit:** Choose from pineapple, mangos, strawberries and a host of other fruits. Eat them fresh, too

- **Hummus:** The vegan's friend! A range of flavours and styles are available. Perfect for picnics, sandwiches and dipping vegetable sticks into

- **Fruit and cereal bars:** Raw fruit bars and baked cereal bars. Just look out for honey

- **Popcorn:** Lots of flavours and brands are vegan – or it's fun to make your own

- **Nuts and seeds:** Always a handy snack to keep in your bag

- **Dark chocolate:** There is iron to be found in dark chocolate, so never feel guilty!

VEGETABLES

Don't hold back here, eat a rainbow every day.

EASY REPLACEMENTS

The simplest way to begin your vegan adventure is to stick to your favourite, tried-and-tested recipes and veganise them by making simple substitutions.

On cereal and in coffee, try different plant milks until you find the ones that suit you best. On toast, pick a dairy-free spread; you will barely notice the difference. And there are many instances where you can swap cheese, ice cream and cream for the dairy-free versions and no one would be any the wiser.

Here's how to veganise a week of popular evening meals.

1. Spaghetti bolognese
Use your favourite recipe, and just use soya mince/soy grounds or lentils instead of the meat. If you'd normally use meat stock, replace with vegetable stock. Use dairy-free margarine or olive oil on the pasta instead of butter. Vegan parmesan can be found in some supermarkets, in health food shops and online.

2. Burgers
There are loads of vegan burgers/patties available; just use an egg-free mayonnaise, which most supermarkets now stock. Ketchup, mustard and pickles are usually already vegan, and you'll find that most bread buns are vegan too

(except those pesky brioche buns, which contain egg). Fancy a cheeseburger? Just use a vegan cheese slice and pick one that melts well.

3. Chilli con carne (or as we call it, chilli *non* carne)
Another simple substitution! Just use soya mince/soy grounds instead of the meat, or use brown lentils if you prefer. If you're using stock, use a vegetable one. Often the pre-mixed chilli spices are vegan. We like to put a little red wine and a dash of cocoa powder in ours.

4. Lasagne
For the meat layer, follow the same pattern as for the bolognese sauce or the chilli, and use soya mince/soy grounds or lentils. For the white sauce, use dairy-free milk and butter. Classicists won't add cheese to a lasagne sauce but if you like it, go ahead and add grated vegan cheese or nutritional yeast flakes. Dried lasagne sheets generally don't contain egg – but fresh ones often do.

5. Fajitas
Replace the meat strips with vegan meat strips! Some of the fajita kits are already vegan, so you need do nothing else except whip up a guacamole; and either leave out the sour cream and cheese or use vegan versions of each. Yes! Vegan sour cream exists.

6. Mac and cheese

Swap the milk for plant milk and the cheese for a melting vegan cheese – you could add nutritional yeast if you like it extra cheesy. That's it!

7. Pizza

If you make the dough yourself, the chances are you're already making a vegan pizza base. If you buy the dough or base, just check that no milk proteins have been added. Add your favourite toppings, including faux ham or salami, and cover with a dairy-free cheese. Make sure the one you buy melts properly.

'I've learned so many new things and cooking techniques that I would never have tried before. Anything you love as a non-vegan you can make vegan.'

Christelle R., Alberta, Canada,
Veganuary Class of 2016

THE ONLY VEGAN IN THE FAMILY

If you're the only one in your household eating vegan at this time, that doesn't have to be a problem, but if you're young and living at home, you may have to clear another hurdle before your vegan adventure can begin. We know that not everyone's families are as supportive as the fledgling vegan might hope, but this is not usually because they like making life hard. It's often because they don't know much about veganism, and they worry about their loved one's health, having to make two separate meals after a long day at work, or how these changes will impact the weekly shopping bill.

If you want to try veganism but are faced with opposition at home, we'd suggest you talk it through as calmly as possible to find out what the reasons are. The sections in this book should help you counter any concerns about health, nutrition and cost, but if the problem lies with having to cook additional meals every day, then it's clear some practicalities will need to be ironed out.

First, if you don't normally help with shopping and cooking this would be a very good time to start. It might be stretching the family bonds just a little too far to expect someone else to do your research, read labels, discover new products and recipes and then cook them for you. Time to step up!

You may find there needs to be a little bargaining at this stage, perhaps something like: *I'll cook a vegan meal for everyone twice a week if you make sure the other meals can be veganised, too.* This doesn't have to be as complex as it might sound! It might be as simple as adding different toppings to a pizza base, or cooking up plant-based sausages, burgers or a pie alongside the meaty ones. So long as the accompaniments are vegan, or can be set aside before someone adds butter or cheese, then this approach shouldn't feel like an extra burden. For something like a stir-fry, simply use the same ingredients split between two pans, then add meat to one and tofu or vegan meaty strips into the other.

Obviously, it will take a little adjusting for everyone, but that's why we suggest people try it for 31 days. That's a great introductory time for everyone to get used to it, and for it to become something like second nature, but if there is still resistance, you might like to throw in some washing-up duties. Some might call that bribery, but if it works . . .

If you're the main cook in your house, or a regular cook, things are usually a lot easier, and the rest of your family will almost certainly be happy with at least some of your veganised versions of family favourite meals. With dishes like chilli and bolognese, there's a good chance that no one will be able to tell the difference anyway. If the others want to add dairy cheese on top when you sprinkle vegan cheese on yours, that's not going to cause any problems.

Even so, there may be times when someone in your household just wants meat or cheese, and there will be no talking them out of it. We can't force others to be vegan, after all. Perhaps you can agree on a set number of vegan meals for everyone each week and then compromise on the others, although whether you will want to cook meat when you're trying out veganism is up to you.

Usually when the household's main cook goes vegan, the whole family tends to eat vegan at home. Chef's rules! But we often find that when people are drawn into plant-based eating because a member of their household is cooking vegan, they find that the new way of eating suits them better than they expected. They are surprised that there are 'meaty' chunks that can be used in casseroles, stews and curries, for example, and 'meat' slices that are great instead of chicken and ham in sandwiches. There are 'chicken' pies, 'beef' pasties, fishless fingers and even vegan haggis – an ever-growing range of great-tasting products that everyone can enjoy.

DOES BEING VEGAN COST MORE?

This is a question that crops up surprisingly often and so Veganuary commissioned Kantar, an independent market research company that specialises in shopping and consumer behaviour, to find out for sure. They found that, on average, plant-based meals eaten at home cost 40 per cent less than meat/fish-based meals. That's quite a saving!

The myth of veganism being expensive probably stemmed from looking at the cost of products in isolation. So, for example, a piece of vegan cheese is likely to cost more than a piece of dairy cheese for lots of reasons, including economy of scale, quality, ingredients and farming subsidies. So, it's easy to point to this one item as 'proof' that veganism is expensive.

What Kantar did is to look at the whole basket of food, not just one product and when we factor in the vegan staples – like pasta, rice, potatoes, beans, tinned tomatoes, lentils and fresh seasonal or frozen veggies – and remove meat and fish, which are probably the most expensive items in the store outside the alcohol aisle, it is easy to see why overall, being vegan is a more affordable way to eat.

It's true, if you rely on convenience foods, you may notice an increase in price, but this does depend on the kinds of products you bought before you were vegan. We conducted a little price comparison exercise ourselves and found that the cost of vegan sausage rolls in one UK supermarket falls right in the middle of the range of the prices for meat-based sausage rolls. And the fishless fingers, while coming towards the top end of the range in terms of cost, are not as expensive as some of the premium fish brands.

If you have traditionally bought foodstuffs at the lower end of the pricing scale, choosing their vegan equivalents might be a greater expense than you are used to, but the overall basket price is still likely to stay the same or come down. And those who used to buy joints of meat, whole organic chickens or premium dairy brands will certainly see the cost of their shopping basket decrease.

No matter what you eat, there are ways to help keep the budget down, including cooking from scratch rather than buying processed or pre-packaged foods, bulk-buying staples such as rice and pasta and cooking up batches of food to freeze for future use.

If you're on a budget, visit the Recipes section of the Veganuary website, where there is a section dedicated to cheap vegan meal ideas. You could also check out Jack Monroe's *Cooking on a Bootstrap* blog, where you'll find lots more delicious and affordable vegan recipes.

And if you're eating out, you'll see that the vegan options on menus are almost always cheaper than the meat-based meals, and there is a good reason for that!

VEGAN OUT
IN THE WORLD

EATING OUT

Once upon a time, a vegan wandering alone and hungry on the high street would have no choice but to buy an apple or a bag of ready salted potato crisps to satisfy the pangs, and wait until they got home before they could eat properly. These days, there is a huge choice of vegan meals on every high street, with restaurant chains vying with one another to offer the widest range and the most exciting dishes. From burgers and burritos to sandwiches and sushi, vegan food is plentiful, varied and just round the corner.

CHAIN RESTAURANTS
In the UK, vegans will find great options at Zizzi, Pizza Express, Wagamama, All Bar One, Domino's, Las Iguanas, Subway, Yo! Sushi, Pret a Manger, Ask, Leon, the Handmade

Burger Company and even Nando's, KFC, McDonald's, Burger King, Gregg's and Toby Carvery.

In the US, look out for options at The Daily Grill, Del Taco, The Cheesecake Factory, Chipotle, Denny's, Jason's Deli, Kona Grill, Little Caesars Pizza, Papa John's, Starbucks, Taco Bell, El Pollo Loco, Veggie Grill, Fatburger, Ike's Sandwiches, Subway and Native Foods.

In Canada, try Teriyaki Experience, Hero Burger, Harvey's, Extreme Pita, Just Falafel, Subway, Magic Oven, Panago Pizza, Chipotle, A&W, Taco Bell, KFC and Tim Hortons.

While in Australia, head to Grill'd, Montezuma's, Sushi Train, Noodle Box, Pizza Hut, Nando's, Sumo Salad, Subway, Indian Brothers, Domino's and Lord of the Fries.

One other international restaurant chain to look out for is Loving Hut – it's 100 per cent vegan, and its restaurants can be found in 35 countries, from England to Australia, from Taiwan to the USA.

VEGGIE AND VEGAN RESTAURANTS

Of course, you're not limited to chain restaurants. There are now so many vegetarian and vegan restaurants, with new ones opening every week, that a host of new eating options will suddenly open up for you. Wherever you are in the world, your best options will be in the cities, but there are plenty of meat-free restaurants opening in smaller towns, too.

From fast food cafes to raw food restaurants to gourmet

plant-based dining, you'll find your best local options at HappyCow.net. Its website and app list thousands of restaurants, cafes and health food stores all over the world, and add news ones regularly. They don't just list specifically vegan restaurants – they list all the restaurants they know of where a vegan meal can be found.

INDEPENDENT RESTAURANTS

With more and more independent restaurants catering for vegans, there is every chance that your favourite eatery will already have – or will happily create – plant-based meals for you.

If you know you're going to a restaurant where you haven't been before – or haven't been since you went vegan – it's wise to call ahead and speak to the chef so you're not left hungry when you visit. It's rare to find a chef who won't prepare a meal for you, and often they relish the challenge of cooking something different from their usual offerings. If you are going to a large get-together, such as a family gathering or a work dinner, it's worth letting the organiser know that you'll personally speak to the venue directly beforehand. That way you can be sure that messages won't get lost or confused, and vital facts won't go missing along the way.

Even if you're not able to call ahead, don't worry; you can still make requests once you're inside the restaurant. By being vegan, you're not being a bore or a burden. You're a customer, and customers make requests *all the time*, for all sorts of reasons, so go ahead and ask for a dish to be altered to suit you. You may be amazed at what a chef can whip up – but if they struggle, you may find that putting a few side dishes together can work surprisingly well.

If you're out with a group and feel a little self-conscious about querying menu items at the table, simply excuse yourself before ordering and have a quiet word with your server. This is also a great way to ask about ingredients, as the waiting staff may need to check with the kitchen, and this can delay the ordering process. You might want to know whether they cook with butter or vegetable oil, if the pasta they use is made with egg, or if the garlic mushrooms can be prepared without cream. And you might find it much easier to ask a few questions when you haven't got (what feels like) a hundred pairs of eyes on you.

A word of warning: although veganism is much more widely understood than ever before, don't assume that all restaurant staff know what it is. Politely explain what you do and don't eat, and take the time to answer their questions. You might say something like, 'I'm vegan, so I don't eat eggs, milk or cheese. I was wondering whether you know if your pizza dough has any milk or eggs in it, and if I can get the Vegetariana pizza without cheese?' You may be the first vegan they've met – so a little patience and politeness will go a long way, and it may just score you a bigger portion. Increasingly, though, serving staff and chefs know exactly what to offer, because they get asked all the time. Besides, all good chefs will know which allergens are in their food – and this handily includes eggs, milk products and shellfish.

INTERNATIONAL CUISINE

Plant-based eaters are usually well fed at restaurants that serve international dishes. From Chinese and Thai to Lebanese, Indian and North African, some delicious and common dishes may already be vegan, or can easily be adapted. When ordering, it's prudent to communicate your vegan needs clearly – as a rule of thumb, a vegetarian diet is well understood across cultures but the term vegan could cause confusion. Stating that you're a *strict vegetarian* and that you do not eat meat, fish, dairy and eggs can often be the best approach to take the stress out of ordering.

Here are some popular favourites and some handy hints on what to watch out for:

Chinese restaurants: spring rolls; bean curd (tofu) in black bean or Szechuan sauce; vegetable dishes, including bean-sprouts; rice or rice noodles.

Watch out for: egg noodles (choose rice noodles instead, often called vermicelli); egg in fried rice; oyster sauce (there's a widely used vegan version made with oyster mushrooms, but some of them do contain real oyster extract – if in doubt, ask to see the bottle); dried shellfish (often used as a garnish on seaweed and other dishes).

Indian restaurants: vegetable samosas, onion bhajis and pakoras; vegetable curries, from biryani to vindaloo; and side dishes, including lentil dhal and bhindi bhaji (okra). Add chapatis, rice, poppadums and chutneys.

Watch out for: yoghurt; ghee (clarified butter – sometimes used instead of oil); paneer (cheese); naan breads which usually contain yoghurt.

Mexican restaurants: totopos (corn chips and tomato dip); guacamole; veggie tacos and tortillas; bean burritos; pozole (corn stew); vegetable or bean chilli; refried beans; potato skins.

Watch out for: cheese and sour cream.

Japanese restaurants: vegetarian gyoza (dumplings); tempura; miso soup; vegetable or avocado rolls; tofu dishes; ramen; vegetable curries.

Watch out for: ponzu sauce (contains tuna); surimi (fish paste); mayonnaise and cream cheese (in westernised veggie sushi); Worcestershire sauce (sometimes called Bulldog sauce – contains anchovies and is used to flavour stews and soups).

Italian restaurants: Pasta pomodoro, arrabiata or Napoli; minestrone soup; vegetarian pizza with vegan cheese or without any cheese; garlic bread (made with olive oil, not butter); olives; salads.

Watch out for: fresh egg pasta; parmesan (stop them before they sprinkle!).

Thai restaurants: Tofu or vegetable satay; tempura; soups and som tam salad; red, green or massaman curries; stir-fried vegetables; coconut rice; noodles.

Watch out for: nam pla (fish sauce) – it can sneak its way into all Thai dishes (particularly curries) but, if the food is freshly prepared, they can leave it out at your request.

Lebanese restaurants: hummus; baba ghanoush (aubergine dip); tabbouleh; falafel; batata harra (spicy potatoes); fava bean dip; okra, beans or aubergines cooked in tomato sauce; flatbreads.

Watch out for: yoghurt; kashk (dairy); labneh (strained yoghurt cheese).

North African restaurants: harira soup; vegetable tagine; couscous; potatoes chermoula; flatbreads; salad.

Watch out for: honey; cheese; yoghurt.

'Through Veganuary, I learned about vegan products I could purchase at regular grocery stores, and also tips for eating out at non-vegan/vegetarian restaurants. After my first month, I was pleasantly surprised at how smooth my transition went. Veganuary was like my personal vegan mentor and I still rely on it for advice and information.'

Britt C., Kansas, US, Veganuary Class of 2017

EATING AT FRIENDS' HOUSES

How do you break the news to your friends and family that the meals they have cooked for you before aren't going to go down so well on your next visit? You don't want to upset, offend, or be a massive pain in their backsides, and you could really do without the questions and jokes that you know are coming your way. For all these reasons, breaking the news to others can feel more daunting than actually going vegan.

The great thing about trying vegan for one month is that it helps others around you accept this change, too. If you say that you're just trying it for 31 days to see how you feel, people will understand much more readily than if you spring on them out of the blue that this former meat addict has gone over to the other side. In our recommended scenario, they are less likely to hit you up with a rapid-fire volley of questions and instead just wonder what to feed you. And that is something you can easily help with.

It's usually a good idea to find out what your host is planning to cook on the occasion of your visit. Perhaps the dish they are planning can easily be made vegan, and you may be able to suggest some tweaks to their menu, such as roasting potatoes in oil rather than goose fat, or using dairy-free butter on the garlic bread. But if not, rather than watch them melt down in sheer panic, why not suggest you bring your own main dish, and match it as closely as possible to theirs? If they'll be eating lasagne, chilli or beef bourguignon, bring a spinach lasagne, a three-bean chilli or a mushroom and red wine casserole. By matching your meals, you won't feel like the odd one out, you will draw less attention to yourself and you'll show the other guests that a vegan meal doesn't have to be so very different from a non-vegan one.

It might be tempting to go ahead and create some mind-blowingly showy vegan dish, with indoor fireworks and sprinkled with gold dust. That would certainly showcase the creativity of veganism; but it might be better to save the theatricals for when you invite people to eat at your home. You don't want to upstage your host. OK, well maybe you do just a little bit.

If your host is happy to adapt a meal for you, you might like to offer to bring a dessert for everyone. This is usually the course where a non-vegan host runs out of steam, and you find yourself sitting in front of a fruit salad which, any way you dress it up, is a) just fruit and b) not a proper dessert (trust us, we're experts on vegan puds).

You'll find amazing recipes online for vegan sticky toffee pudding, treacle tart, chocolate torte, Key lime pie, brownies, pavlovas and many other popular desserts. By bringing your favourite vegan treat, you'll take some pressure off your host, add to your own vegan cookery repertoire and show off vegan food. You'll also be sure to get a great dessert!

What about Christmas, Thanksgiving, weddings and birthdays? The same advice applies: find out what's being made, suggest a few tweaks so you can enjoy as many of the dishes as possible and offer to bring anything else. If the food you make looks amazing, your host may just borrow your recipes for next time.

DEALING WITH FAMILY AND FRIENDS*

For some new vegans, breaking the news to family and friends will provoke one of three reactions. First, your loved ones might find this the most hilarious thing that has *ever* happened. You'll have to put up with some truly original witticisms about wimpy vegans, your transition to a hippy lifestyle and eating nothing but grass. We know. Hilarious.

They may also become instant nutrition experts and warn you of the myriad ways in which you are likely to waste away. Fear not, we'll be coming to nutrition shortly.

But what is equally likely to happen is that you, as a fresh-faced new vegan, brimming with enthusiasm, will immediately start trying to persuade all your friends to join you in this plant-based adventure.

Let's take a look at each of these scenarios, starting with your terrifically funny friends. If you think they're likely to make you the butt of a million jokes before they just accept you've decided to try vegan, you could try *not* telling them for a few weeks, so when they start up with the tired old clichés, you can respond: *That's old news. I've been vegan for ages and you didn't even notice.* That might just take the wind out of their sails.

---

* This advice can be extended to colleagues, school mates and that guy you bump into at the gym – all of whom are bound to have an opinion at some point

But if it's just your turn to be the target of their banter, rising to it certainly won't make it go away. You'll just have to laugh along and take it on the chin. In time, they'll lose interest, especially if they see you eating some great food, and notice you're kicking their butts at the gym or out on the pitch. Besides, for better or worse, these are the people who have stood by you in hard times. They are your friends for a reason and there isn't much you can do to shake off family. But what is interesting is that, in our experience, those that laugh loudest are often the most interested. Give them a little space to ask the questions they are probably bursting to know and see how many of them in time follow your lead. You might be surprised.

Onto scenario two: the instant expert. This is something all new vegans will probably have to face at some point. It will likely start with *Where do you get your protein?* and, depending on the headlines they've read most recently, could also take in B12, choline, omega-3 or the subject of any other scare story that serves as media clickbait. It may be they are not being mischievous, but are genuinely worried, although for some, it could be a way of justifying their decision not to become vegan, too. Whatever their motivation, it is wise for your own health to know a bit about nutrition, and you'll find all the basics in the next chapter. But at this stage, rest assured: it is perfectly possible to get every nutrient you need on a vegan diet.

Now, let's turn to the other possible outcome of your announcement. You could be feeling so great on your plant-based diet – sleeping better, looking better, full of energy and with a clear conscience. You may even be feeling a little smug about it all. That's OK. When we switch to a diet that is good news for animals, great for our health, helps feed the world and protects the planet, we can all get a little exuberant, even evangelical. A word to the wise: self-righteousness rarely goes down well, and nor does haranguing people about all the reasons why they are wrong to eat animal products.

If you don't like being lectured, or having your faults, inconsistencies and personality flaws pointed out, you can be sure that others feel the same. The people in your life will be much more responsive to the benefits of eating plant-based foods when you're calm and rational, not when you're parked outside their house with a banner and a megaphone.

What does work is being a great example, and a nice person. Some of what you learn as a vegan may have become so obvious to you that it's easy to forget there was ever a time when you didn't know it, but for your friends and family there is a lot to take in. And the things that horrify us most can be the hardest to accept. It's a difficult thing, after all, to accept that the diet we've always chosen has an impact on the world's hungriest or causes suffering to millions of animals. If you blame others for these things, the shutters will come down, and they will tell you where to go. Exactly as you would if they had done the same to you.

Patience and acceptance is key. Even when people hear about all the reasons that being vegan is wonderful, they'll still worry about what they will eat. Inside, we might be screaming *WHAT ABOUT THE ANIMALS?* or *YOU ARE KILLING THE PLANET!* But we should never forget these legitimate concerns about missing out on favourite foods. If we're honest, it may well have been the thing that stopped us going vegan sooner, too. People can be scared of change. That's normal, and OK. It can take time for someone to understand the issues, be reassured and also be in a position to make the choice to go vegan. Be kind and tolerant, and accept that – although you can educate and influence people – what they eat is their choice, as much as what you eat is yours.

Of course, however tolerant you are, at times you will face negative attitudes – others may even set out to trip you up and it can be upsetting. Accusations of hypocrisy could be thrown at you for a whole host of reasons, from buying bottled water to taking a flight or even driving a car. It's a common misconception that your new vegan status should go hand in hand with shunning a whole catalogue of modern lifestyle choices. Your go-to response could be something like 'Being vegan reduces my impact on the planet significantly – but of course there are other ways I could improve.'

Similarly, don't be made to feel guilty about your pre-vegan choices. Whilst dietary change can be immediate, you're not expected to rush out and replace all your worldly possessions so your wallet might still be leather and you may still wear your favourite woollen jumper. That doesn't make you a hypocrite but sadly, not everyone understands that doing what you can is better than doing nothing at all. A good approach is to slowly replace your belongings with vegan versions as and when you need to, and you can explain that throwing or giving away non-vegan items does nothing to protect the animals affected and could lead to even more landfill.

VEGAN TRAVELLING

You've become something of an expert on the range of vegan goodies that can be found in your local shops and restaurants, but what happens when you travel further afield? Depending on where your travels take you, things might be trickier. In some countries, meat is at the centre of every meal, and is also in the sauce, and mixed in with the vegetables too. So, it's wise to undertake a little research before you leave your home, to find out what the region's delicacies are and what they're made from. Search online for vegans who live there or have visited the area and see what tips they might have for you.

Of course, it's also possible that you will be surprised to find there are dozens of vegetarian or vegan restaurants at your chosen location, or at least a few where you can find some delicious vegan options. HappyCow.net is a great place to find this out. Lots of people become vegan tourists, planning their holidays around the locations with the most vegan restaurants, and there's no shame in that! Food is an important part of a holiday and, while there are many cities where you'll find exceptional vegan food within a fascinating location, these are some of the cities that crop up over and over as the vegans' favourites.

1. Berlin, Germany
2. Melbourne, Australia
3. Tel Aviv, Israel
4. New York City, USA
5. Toronto, Canada
6. Chennai, India
7. London, UK
8. Taipei, Taiwan
9. Warsaw, Poland
10. Barcelona, Spain

As for accommodation, wherever you're going, check beforehand that the hotel or guesthouse can cater for you. Most hotels can offer a basic breakfast – fresh fruit, bread and jam, tea and coffee, cereals and plant-based milks. Others may be able to whip you up something else on request. But if they aren't able to provide a main meal and you're worried about finding suitable fare in local restaurants, again, ask for advice from one of the many vegan social media groups online. There may be someone who has been there or who lives there and has valuable insider knowledge.

In areas where vegan restaurants are hard to find, you'll still always find vegan ingredients, so if you're still drawing a blank, you may prefer to go self-catering.

Or maybe you'd like to make things super easy on yourself, take a complete break from cooking and instead be fully pampered, in which case check out the growing range of exclusively vegetarian and vegan hotels. You'll find them all over the world. You may even like to go on a fully vegan cruise or a dedicated vegan adventure or activity-based holiday. All these things exist so the world is very much your oyster mushroom.

To throw yourself fully into the Vegan Traveller experience, it's best to learn (or at least carry with you) some basic phrases: *I'm vegan* and *I don't eat meat, fish, milk or eggs* are good places to start. The Vegan Society in the UK produces a Vegan Passport app, which offers useful phrases in 78 languages including Hausa, Igbo, Xhosa and Zulu, and images for where language still falls short. They also produce a hard-copy phrasebook you can pull out when needed.

Online translation services might also save the day, although they are not always 100 per cent reliable. (We certainly *hope* there were no fried ravens in those Slovenian chocolate wafers we ate.) And therein lies a valuable lesson. We are more likely to make a mistake when travelling than we are at home. We may be reading labels in another language, relying on translations or just hoping that the charades we are acting out can be understood. Most of us have eaten something we *think* is vegan but we can't be sure. Don't sweat it too much. It's not about perfection. It's about doing our best.

Nonetheless, it's a good idea to be prepared. There's

nothing worse than trawling the streets with your stomach growling while you search for a vegan restaurant you know is there somewhere but can't find. Make sure you pack some snacks in your luggage to see you through any such grumpy periods. Cereal bars, dried fruits and nuts and a chocolate bar or two should be packed alongside your swim kit and sunscreen. Hopefully you'll bring them home again, but you'll be glad to know you have them as back-up.

NUTRITION
IN A NUTSHELL

So, you want to try being vegan but there's someone in your life telling you it can't be good for you, that you'll get sick, be anaemic and protein-deficient, lose weight and probably expire before the week is out. It's nice that they worry, but they really shouldn't. You can get all the nutrients you need on a vegan diet – but you should be aware that with so many convenient plant-based products out there, is it also a little too easy to be a junk food vegan. As with any diet, it's essential we get enough of the right nutrients and limit the stuff we all know to be bad for us. Here are a few things to look out for.

PROTEIN

It's very hard to be protein-deficient, and yet this is the nutrient that people seem to worry about most. This may be because of a common misconception that you have to consume meat to get enough protein. You don't! Just because there is protein in meat doesn't mean it doesn't exist anywhere else. In fact, vegans simply do what cows, pigs, sheep and chickens do: we go directly to the source. Green vegetables (the superstars are kale, broccoli, seaweed and peas), beans and pulses (lentils, lima, edamame, pinto, black and tofu), grains (rice, pasta, quinoa and bulgur) and nuts (Brazils, peanuts, cashews, almonds, pistachios, pine nuts, walnuts and nut butters) are all excellent sources of protein.

Protein is needed for healthy enzymes, hormones and antibodies, and to build and repair muscles, but how much of it do we need? Guidelines vary depending on gender, age, activity levels and even where you live, since different countries' governments give different recommended intakes. But, as an example, we'll take a 30-year-old woman, not pregnant, who is active, engaging in one hour per day of walking or jogging, or 30 minutes of running. Her requirement is 47g of protein a day. For an active man of similar age, the requirement is 56g.

If she were to eat peanut butter on toast for breakfast, one hummus and falafel wrap and a shepherd's pie (made with soya mince) for dinner, she would easily exceed her required protein intake. And that's before she adds in the dairy-free milk she puts in her tea, some bread with her soup, the green vegetables with her dinner (there is 4g in a serving of broccoli and 5g in peas), or the soya milkshake, cereal bar or handful of nuts she has as a snack.

These are the protein levels in some everyday vegan meals:

Nutrition in a Nutshell

BREAKFAST
Peanut butter on toast (2 pieces) 15g
Typical cereal with soya yoghurt and a handful of nuts 13g
Porridge/oatmeal with a sprinkle of almonds or seeds 12g

LUNCH
Three-bean salad wrap (2 wraps) 18g
Beans on toast (2 pieces) 17g
Hummus and falafel wrap (3 falafels, one wrap) 15g

DINNER
Tofu and vegetable stir-fry with brown rice 32g
Veggie sausages* (2), potato and peas 26g
Shepherd's pie, made with soya mince 20g

Other great protein-rich vegan foods to look out for are seitan, which has an incredible 30g of protein per serving, tempeh, quinoa, and cashew or almond nut butters. But there is protein in almost all foods, including pasta, potatoes and vegetables, and so it's actually really hard to go short of it with a balanced vegan diet. Bodybuilders looking to increase their intake for significant muscle gain can choose one of the many vegan protein powders on the market, and incorporate it into their diets via protein shakes or balls.

If anyone suggests that plant-eaters can't be muscular and powerful, ask them to think about where elephants, rhinos,

* Not all veggie sausages have high protein levels; check the label

hippos, mountain gorillas, oxen, water buffalo and bison get their protein from. The answer is, of course, plants. Just try telling a gorilla she's protein-deficient.

CALCIUM

In the same way that some people think protein and meat are synonymous, it's common to hear people conflate calcium with milk. We absolutely need calcium for strong bones (along with its super sidekick vitamin D, which helps us to absorb it) but we don't need to drink cows' milk to get it.

Most of the calcium in our bodies can be found in our bones, so if we don't consume enough of it our bodies will use up this store, and that can weaken our bones. The loss of too much calcium can lead to osteoporosis later in life, so it's important to ensure that we get a good supply.

You can boost your intake with beans (especially black turtle beans, kidney beans and soya beans), kale, collards, watercress, okra, broccoli, sweet potato and butternut squash. (Spinach has loads of calcium but it's poorly absorbed due to the oxalic acid in the leaves.) You can also snack on dried figs and almonds, and include some calcium-set tofu in your meals.

If you're buying plant milks, look for brands that are fortified with calcium, and the same goes for yoghurts, too. There's no need to restrict yourself to health foods in the quest for calcium – even delicious vegan milkshakes are often calcium-rich.

As for vitamin D, there's no better source than the sun,

and 15 minutes of exposure a day during spring, summer and autumn should suffice so long as your face, hands and arms are exposed. But older or overweight people, those who don't spend time outside, and those who live in northern latitudes or who have darker skin,[1] could be at greater risk of deficiency and may wish to choose dairy-free butters, breakfast cereals and breads that are already fortified with it. You may also want to consider a supplement. This is wise for everyone, no matter their diet, because a lack of vitamin D is surprisingly common, and can affect muscles and mood as well.[2] In the UK, the government recommends everyone take a vitamin D supplement in the winter as the sun does not contain enough UVB radiation for our skin to make vitamin D.

While we're talking bone health, it's wise to avoid smoking, as this is a risk factor for osteoporosis. We should also do regular weight-bearing exercise (making you work against gravity), such as walking, running, dancing, playing tennis or football or lifting weights in the gym.

IRON

Iron is needed to make the red blood cells that carry oxygen around the body. If we don't get enough, there's a risk of iron-deficiency anaemia. That could be the source of the outdated 'pale, tired vegetarian' myth. The truth is that iron-deficiency anaemia is commonplace across all diets, and particularly in those who menstruate. For this reason, the recommended intake for women is significantly higher than for men: 14.8mg a day in the UK as opposed to 8.7mg for men,[3] and 18mg a day in the US as opposed to 8mg for men.[4] Pregnant women will need more, and a supplement might be considered easiest.

The good news is that women who eat a plant-based diet do not appear to be any more at risk of iron deficiency than those who eat meat, and there is no reason why any vegan should struggle to get enough iron so long as their diet is healthy and balanced.

It's easy to start the day with an iron boost. Many breakfast cereals are fortified with iron, so check to see if your favourite vegan one is. Oats are also a good source of iron, so eating porridge or oatmeal will get you off to a racing start. If you're a man and add a handful of dried fruit to your breakfast and a sprinkle of pumpkin seeds on top, you may have reached your required daily intake before you've even changed out of your pyjamas.

For lunch and dinner, we should remember that pulses are our pals.

Soybeans	8.6mg per cup
Lentils	5.4 – 6.5mg per cup
Peas including chickpeas/garbanzo	2.5 – 4.6mg per cup
Beans including kidney beans	3.4 – 6.5mg of iron per cup[5]

Other sources to help you hit your target include: dark chocolate, blackstrap molasses and black treacle, tofu, tempeh, quinoa and dark leafy green vegetables like watercress and kale. Almonds, Brazil nuts and sesame seeds also contain a useful amount of iron.

Two little tips to help boost iron absorption: eat foods that contain vitamin C and don't drink coffee or tea (either black or green) with a meal.[6]

Now, while getting the right amount of iron is obviously good, ingesting too much iron is actually pretty bad. Luckily, our bodies are great at regulating iron – if we don't have enough circulating around our bodies, our intestines take more of it from our food. If there's too much, they take less. Interestingly, research suggests that our clever intestines can only do this effectively with iron from plants. Iron from meat can't be regulated so easily, and researchers are starting to raise questions about whether too much iron from meat is linked to cancer and cardiovascular disease.[7]

OMEGA-3

Fats are our friends. We need fatty acids to ensure the proper functioning of all our tissues, so it's great news that our bodies are able to make almost all the fatty acids we need. There are two, however, that we cannot make and therefore it's absolutely essential that we eat them. For this reason they are called 'essential' fatty acids. They're known as omega-3 and omega-6.

Deficiency is associated with kidney disease, heart disease, Alzheimer's, osteoarthritis, bowel disease and depression.[8] So, where can we get these essential acids?

Omega-6 can be found plentifully in leafy vegetables, seeds, nuts, grains and most vegetable oils. It is very easy to get sufficient omega-6 on a balanced diet – but this is where things start to get a little tricky. In all people, regardless of their diet, omega-6 acids compete with omega-3 acids for use in the body. So we need to pay attention and ensure we are eating sufficient omega-3 on a daily basis. Small amounts can be found in nuts, seeds, soya products, beans, vegetables and whole grains but the best sources of omega-3 are:

- Leafy vegetables, such as Brussels sprouts, kale, spinach and salad leaves
- Walnuts
- Rapeseed oil
- Ground flaxseed[9]
- Flaxseed oil
- Soybeans and tofu[10]
- Black lentils, also known as urad dal and mungo beans (not to be confused with mung beans)[11]

Ground flaxseed? Have you ever heard anything more stereotypically vegan in all your life?! Don't despair. These ground-up seeds are quite common, and can be found in most supermarkets and health food shops. Add them to smoothies or muffin recipes or sprinkle them on your breakfast cereal and you won't even notice that you're getting a massive health boost. Eating a handful of walnuts as a snack will go a long way in ensuring you're getting enough omega-3 each day.

If you're still worried, physician and author Dr Michael Greger recommends taking 250mg of pollutant-free long-chain omega-3s in the form of supplements, two or three times per week. These are obtained from algae – the same place that fish get their omega-3 from, and if we choose these instead, the cod will get to keep their livers.

VITAMIN B12

This little vitamin can be quite elusive. One study revealed that 1 in 12 British women between the ages of 19 and 39 are deficient despite consuming the recommended intake[12] and deficiency can bring some pretty unpleasant symptoms. So let's all agree to get enough B12.

This vitamin is present in animal products, but it isn't made by the animals themselves; it's created by the bacteria that live inside them. Since vegans don't want to eat the animals – or their delicious bacteria – we can get B12 by instead eating yeast extracts, nutritional yeast flakes and breakfast cereals and plant-based milks that are fortified with it. Check the packaging to be sure your chosen brand contains B12. The more we spread out our intake, the less we need to consume, so ideally we'd eat three portions a day of B12-fortified foods. But our hectic lifestyles often make it difficult to ensure we are getting enough B12 from our food, so to be safe we recommend taking a supplement. They can be taken in tablet form or in a spray and the recommended amount is 1.5 micrograms per day.[13]

It's not just vegans who need to keep an eye on their B12 intake. People who suffer from Crohn's or lupus, or who drink heavily, are at risk of being deficient. Since the risk of deficiency increases with age, the advice given in the US is for everyone over the age of 50 to get their B12 from fortified foods or a supplement regardless of their dietary choices.[14]

IODINE

Iodine is needed to make the thyroid hormones that keep our cells healthy and control our metabolism. Adults need 150mcg a day, except when pregnant or breastfeeding, then we require 200mcg.[15] Although we are warned against consuming too much iodine, in Japan, which has among the highest consumption of iodine in the world, intake is thought to be in the region of 1,000-3,000mcg a day – up to 20 times the amount recommended in the UK.[16]

Non-vegans in the West tend to get their iodine from milk but it's not a natural component of dairy. In fact, the majority of iodine in milk is due to contamination with the iodine-based disinfectant used to clean the cows' teats and the milking machinery.[17] Mmmm. Tasty.

Iodine is also found in fish and eggs but where does this leave vegans? We can get a little from nuts, fruits and vegetables, but it is unlikely to be sufficient and in any case it is impossible to know how much these contain as it depends on the composition of the soil they were grown in. So, what to do? The best source of iodine for vegans is seaweed but again, levels vary widely, depending on the type, the sea they were harvested from, and whether they are cooked.[18] If you like the taste of seaweed, you could incorporate some into your diet regularly, as is the case in Japan, and you are unlikely to go short of it.

Another option is to use iodised salt instead of table salt or sea salt. Many people find their blood pressure drops when they become vegan,[19] so this may be an appropriate option. But for those with high blood pressure, a supplement could be the right way to go.

GETTING IT RIGHT

It's entirely possible to eat a nutritionally balanced vegan diet and thrive as a result. But it's also possible to get it wrong. If we live on fizzy drinks, fries and chocolate, we might be vegan but we shouldn't expect to stay healthy for long. As a vegan, you are likely to be challenged about your diet by family and friends who show their concern by becoming nutritional experts. Learning about nutrition will help you put their minds at rest; but most importantly, it will give you the best chance of optimal health.

There is an app we recommend that can help you hit all your targets – Dr Greger's Daily Dozen is available for iPhone and Android, and lets you track quite easily the foods you should aim to eat every day. If you're in any doubt, or have additional health conditions, always consult a medical professional.

VEGAN KIDS

What we feed ourselves is a matter of personal choice but when it comes to making decisions for our children, the responsibility can feel overwhelming, especially if you are considering bringing up your children vegan or if you are hoping to change their diet in line with your own. There is a lot to consider but we need to reassure you straight off the bat. It is perfectly possible to raise a happy, healthy vegan child, and millions of families around the world are doing just that. But there are things you need to know, and here we aim to provide some useful information and a few pointers to get you started.

SHOULD WE BRING UP OUR KIDS VEGAN?

That is for every parent to decide and while for some it is a straightforward question with a very clear answer, for others it can be a difficult decision to make. It's not just about being confident that you will get the nutrition right, important as that is. There are also concerns about children fitting in with their peers as they grow, not missing out on big occasions, and knowing you will have to give difficult and upsetting answers to some inevitable questions, such as 'Why are we vegan?' and 'Why do my friends eat animals?'

At the same time, we know that most children do not want to hurt animals and have a profound sense of justice. It's clear that if they knew what meat was and what animals went through for it to end up on their plates, many, perhaps most, would want none of it. This brings us up against a regularly voiced criticism that in bringing up vegan children, you are inflicting your choices or beliefs on them.

But isn't that what every parent does for their child? Every parent chooses what to feed their child, at least in the early months and years, and we might just as well say that people are inflicting meat-eating on their children. But, of course, we don't see it that way. All parents are doing their best, and we know this can be a tricky subject to navigate.

In terms of nutrition, the British Dietetic Association has confirmed that a well-planned vegan diet is suitable for all stages of life, including pregnancy, breastfeeding and child-hood.[1] And beyond nutrition, we would invite you to consider the wider lessons that veganism teaches children: compassion, standing up for what is right, caring for our planet and others, and sharing the world's resources – all lessons we teach our children anyway.

The essence of being vegan means we really live by those principles.

In the end, whatever you decide is right for you, we urge you to do your own research, find reputable voices and resources, ignore the misleading and unreliable, and try not to be swayed by click-bait headlines.

'Well-planned vegetarian and vegan diets with appropriate attention to specific nutrient components can provide a healthy alternative lifestyle at all stages of fetal, infant, child and adolescent growth.'

Canadian Paediatric Society,
Community Paediatrics Committee[2]

VEGAN PREGNANCY AND BREASTFEEDING

If you are eating a balanced vegan diet, you'll also be eating healthily for two (or more) when pregnant, but still there are a couple of things to look out for as a vegan.

During pregnancy, it is important to be aware of calorific intake, especially during the second and third trimesters when gastric capacity decreases as the baby takes up more room.[3][4] On top of that, in the third trimester additional calories are needed – NICE (The National Institute for Health and Care Excellence in the UK) recommends 200 additional calories a day for the last three months.[5] Achieving this could be an issue if a typical wholefood, high-fibre diet fills you up before the required calorific intake has been achieved. If this is likely, researchers suggest consuming fruit and vegetable juices, peeled beans, and high-protein, high-energy, fibre-free foods such as soya milk, tofu, and soya yoghurt.[6] Anyone struggling to gain the weight they are expected to gain at any point in the pregnancy should consider a consultation with a plant-based nutritionist.

The second issue to be aware of is the increased need for certain nutrients during pregnancy. The official advice about daily intakes varies from country to country but in most cases, it requires little change to an already healthy diet,[7] as absorption efficiency also changes during pregnancy. Nonetheless, let us reassure you about some of the key nutrients, and examine more closely others you may be advised to increase.

SUFFICIENT FROM A BALANCED HEALTHY DIET

- Iron requirements increase during pregnancy and more is needed as the pregnancy advances, but since iron is not lost through menstruation and because more iron is absorbed, the recommended intake remains the same.[8] However, ensuring a good supply of iron-rich foods in the diet is certainly beneficial.

- Zinc. Research suggests that those who don't eat animal products may consume less zinc and although their blood levels of zinc tend to be lower, they also tend to remain in the normal range.[9] Like iron, zinc requirements increase during pregnancy, but efficiency of absorption also increases.[10]

- Vitamin B12. It is not necessary to increase your B12 consumption during pregnancy, but it is essential you are getting sufficient every day, pregnant or not. The safest way to do that is to take a supplement.

- Calcium. During pregnancy, the efficiency of calcium absorption increases so there is no need to increase the amount of calcium in the diet.[11] However, vegans can fall short of calcium if they are not careful and so it is essential to keep an eye on this nutrient.

- More protein is needed during pregnancy, but most people get sufficient in their diets anyway. The NHS advice is to eat protein-rich foods daily during pregnancy to be sure to cover the additional requirements.[12]

- Iodine. Again, more is needed during pregnancy so make sure you are getting sufficient in your diet. As we know, getting a reliable source of iodine can be tricky so supplementing may be the best option at any time, including pregnancy.

ONES TO WATCH
The British Dietetic Association recommends two supplements during pregnancy: folic acid and vitamin D.

- Folate / folic acid. Since folate is found naturally in many vegetables, vegans should be getting plenty. Good sources include broccoli, Brussels sprouts, leafy green vegetables, peas, chickpeas, kidney beans and fortified breakfast cereals. Still, it is advised that those wishing to get pregnant and those in the first 12 weeks of pregnancy take a daily 400 mcg folic acid supplement.[13]

- Vitamin D. The advice for pregnancy is the same as the general advice: that it's not always possible to get sufficient from the sun and so it is recommended that all pregnant women take 10 mcg of vitamin D daily. Those who have darker skin or reduced exposure to sunlight should take 25 mcg of vitamin D daily.[14]

FOOD TO AVOID IN PREGNANCY
There is quite a list to foods to avoid because they are potentially harmful to you and/or the unborn baby.[15] They include: certain cheeses such as brie, camembert, soft blue cheeses

and any made from unpasteurised milk; raw and under-cooked meats; anything with liver; all pates; meats from 'game' animals, such as goose, pheasant or partridge; raw or undercooked eggs and certain fish including all raw shellfish.

Have you noticed what these have in common? Vegans can pretty much relax! (Though the advice is also to avoid caffeine, alcohol and some herbal teas.)

BREASTFEEDING

If you're already supplementing with vitamins B12, iodine and vitamin D, the advice is to continue to do that throughout breastfeeding, but you should be able to get all the other nutrients you need quite easily on a balanced vegan diet.[16]

At the time of writing, there are no approved vegan formulas for newborns in the UK or US (though there are elsewhere in the world) but there are non-dairy, nutritionally complete soya formulas available,[17] with the only non-vegan ingredient being the vitamin D that is derived from the lanolin in sheep's wool.

Please don't be tempted to make your own plant milk for your baby. It may not be nutritionally appropriate or sterile.

NUTRITION FOR KIDS

Introducing foods to your child as a vegan has all the same challenges and joys as for any other parent. And, according to Claire McCarthy, MD, Senior Faculty Editor at Harvard

Health Publishing, there are two issues that vegan parents should learn about and plan for: calories and protein. Plant-based foods tend to have fewer calories than animal foods, which is what makes them so great for adults. But children and teens must get sufficient calories which may not be possible if they fill up on high-fibre foods. The advice is to use nuts, nut butters, avocados, soya products and granola to add calories as they grow.[18]

As for protein, it is essential to meet the requirements as . . . news flash . . . children grow fast, and they need that protein to meet those growth needs and to provide energy. As with calories, the amount of protein a child needs depends on their age and size but can be met with nuts, nut butters, legumes, soya products and cereals.[19] Research shows that soya protein can meet needs as effectively as animal protein,[20] but it is always best to feed them a variety of protein-rich foods.

There is not space in this book to set out full nutritional profiles for children of every age, but that information is readily available. Here we just wish to reassure you that a varied diet can meet all their needs but – as with your own diet – there are a few nutrients we would do well to keep an eye on: iron, calcium, vitamins B12 and D, essential fatty acids (omega-3 and -6), zinc, and iodine.

There is limited scientific data about the impact of a vegan diet on children's growth but what there is suggests no significant impact on their height at five years,[21] or in adolescence.[22]

Researchers from the Nutrition Unit at the University of Zaragoza in Spain together with the Department of Paediatrics at Imperial College London state: *'Adequate and realistic meal planning guidelines should not be difficult to achieve, thanks to the increasing number and availability of natural and fortified vegan foods, which can help children to meet all their nutrient requirements.'*[23]

So please be reassured. Researchers tend to agree that: *'A completely plant-based diet is suitable during pregnancy, lactation, infancy, and childhood, provided that it is well-planned.'*[24]

RECOMMENDED READING
Nourish by Reshma Shah MD, MPH and Brenda Davies RD
Disease-Proof Your Child by Joel Fuhrman MD

CASE STUDY

LESLEY JEAVONS: RAISING A VEGAN CHILD TO ADULTHOOD
We decided to raise Aidan vegan, as we're vegan so why wouldn't we?

We certainly didn't have any concerns at all about the healthiness of his diet. The only concern we did have was the opinion of others, but we'd had to deal with that ourselves since we became vegan so we weren't too worried.

We didn't have any challenges from medical professionals. Living in Brighton, midwives and doctors were probably more aware of vegans than in some other towns and cities back in 2001 and would have had first-hand experience of vegan families. Babies and young children have regular check-ups and it was evident that Aidan had a varied healthy diet, was a good eater and was thriving.

As he grew, we spoke to other parents so if he was going to a friend's for dinner or a sleepover they would make a meal that Aidan could eat and wasn't alien to them, such as Linda McCartney sausages or a veggie chilli, and they would buy soya milk for Aidan to have the same breakfast cereals that they did.

Aidan went through school having packed lunches and though there would be some vegan options at birthday parties, we'd always send him off with some extra bits, especially cake. Often at school, kids would bring in sweets or cakes for their birthdays. If we knew about a birthday in advance we'd always make sure that the school had something different to give Aidan, and if it was sprung on us and he was quite sad to have missed out – which was the only time he ever struggled with being vegan for a short time – we always ensured we got him something just as good or even better so that he didn't mind missing out at the time. It's made him good at delayed gratification!

When he reached his teenage years he would go out to eat with his mates for a pizza, and at Japanese or Chinese restaurants, and Aidan could easily eat vegan alongside them without it being an issue.

Aidan is now 20 and we would imagine that any of the

minor issues we faced 20 years ago would be much less of an issue nowadays. You'd be hard-pushed to find a restaurant chain doing birthday parties that doesn't have vegan options on the menu or a supermarket not selling vegan sweets or cakes. And whereas we often used to be the only vegans some people knew, nowadays it seems everyone knows another vegan so it's been 'normalised' and that makes things easier still.

People can be quite judgemental of other people's lifestyle choices and you can be damned either way: give your child only wholefoods and you're a killjoy; give them junk food and you're looked down upon as being no better than anyone else (even though you never implied you were!). So I'd recommend trying to give your child the most varied diet you can that helps them integrate with their peers, but doesn't compromise on vegan ethics.

As Aidan is a life vegan, when he first learnt that people ate animals he found it quite alien, distressing and hard to understand. He's very empathetic, compassionate and a huge animal lover and has never swayed from being vegan; he sees it is as weird to eat any animal as it would be to eat one of our cats.

NAVIGATING SCHOOL MEALS AND OUTINGS

Feeding your child vegan at home is one thing; managing what they eat out of it is another. There are bound to be mistakes and challenges along the way so it's good to be reminded that veganism is 'a philosophy and way of living which seeks to exclude—*as far as is possible and practicable*—all forms of exploitation of, and cruelty to, animals for food, clothing or any other purpose.'

Some schools are better than others in providing animal-free meals, so discussing your requirements with the caterers or the head teacher as soon as possible is essential. In most countries, there is no legislation that requires schools to provide vegan options, but many will do so.

We hear of some real success stories – of varied, delicious, nutritious foods being provided but there are inevitably some less-positive outcomes, too. In the UK, The Vegan Society can help parents who are struggling to get vegan food for their child. In the US, the Physicians Committee for Responsible Medicine works with school districts, governments, students and parents to bring plant-based foods into schools. Nonetheless, for some parents, the most practical way to ensure a healthy, varied diet is to provide a packed lunch.

School outings can add another layer of complexity and may require a phone call to the school and / or the destination to see what food will be available there, and again a packed lunch may be the better option. Of course, there is another discussion to be had about the outing itself, and whether you – as a compassionate vegan – support it. Zoos and other similar destinations can test your ethical boundaries, with parents needing to weigh up the wellbeing and positive integration of their child with their own views on keeping wild animals in captivity. These are issues that may test you but then no one ever said raising children was going to be a breeze!

Whatever feels right to you is the right course of action but wherever possible, we'd recommend a collaborative approach, working with schools and caterers, and calling on support from national organisations where needed.

BIRTHDAY PARTIES

Yes, birthday parties can be super stressful. How you navigate them will be up to you and your child. Some older children – those who understand and support the reasons for being vegan – will not want to eat anything that contains animal products and will ask all the right questions themselves. But still, you won't want them to miss out. So, speaking with the host beforehand means you may be able to provide like-for-like options, which will ensure your child gets the same sugar rush as everyone else without the animal products.

If the party is held at a fast-food restaurant, there are increasingly good options for vegans available there, and your child should find something to eat. But if they're left disappointed, you may wish to treat them at the end of the day to something special – either out at a local restaurant that you know creates fantastic child-friendly food or by cooking them their favourite meal at home.

For very young children or those who do not yet fully understand veganism, you may need to be their eyes and ears. But again, it is a balancing act. Parties are supposed to be fun, a time of great enjoyment, of friendship and social play. The last thing you want is to turn the event into a series of massive public disappointments.

It bears repeating that all vegans make mistakes, and it is all the more likely that young children will do so. It's OK. We'll just keep working towards a world where all birthday cakes are vegan.

ANSWERING THEIR QUESTIONS

Kids ask a lot of questions, but how do we tell them why we choose to be vegan when the reason may be related to the traumatic exploitation of animals? Many parents say that gentle, simple honesty is the best approach.

Because meat comes from an animal and we don't want to hurt our animal friends – may be sufficient to start with. But the questions will keep coming, and you may need to gently drip through information, keeping back anything that is likely to cause distress. It may be these conversations lead to talking about sexual reproduction and death sooner than you might have liked. But keeping the responses brief and to the point, and emphasising that *we don't eat animals because we love them*, may be the best approach for young children. If you care for any animals at home you can explain that *we wouldn't want anyone to hurt Fido/Fluffy and cows and chickens are no different.*

A trip to an animal sanctuary if there is one nearby can be a great starting point for these conversations. There, your child can meet pigs, sheep, ducks, chickens and cows, and see for themselves just how wonderful they are. It will be a memorable day out and will help your child understand the commitment you have made to a compassionate life.

Complexities may come when they start to ask why their friends, cousins, grandparents and teachers eat animals. Maybe even a parent does, too. They may be upset and ask, *'Don't they care about animals?'* Obviously, you don't want to change the way they feel about the people they love but it may be a question that deep down you are itching to ask, too.

It's OK to say, 'Everyone makes their own choices. We choose to be vegan but not everyone thinks the same way as us. Maybe they just don't know what we know about how amazing animals are.'

Thankfully, in recent years there has been a wealth of beautiful books written and illustrated for vegan children. Some explain why we choose to be vegan; others are stories of animals. Many authors of mainstream books deal beautifully with animals and compassion, without explicitly being vegan books because almost all kids love animals. And if the reality is explained to them gently and sensitively, most completely understand the choice you have made, even if they might waiver when that non-vegan birthday cake is brought out.

We would like to thank the following doctors for providing advice on this chapter:

Dr S. K. Sethi
MD FRCPCH MPH DIBLM
CONSULTANT PAEDIATRICIAN
BOARD CERTIFIED LIFESTYLE PHYSICIAN

Dr Miriam Martinez-Biarge
PAEDIATRICIAN

VEGAN FOR SPORTS

Not only is it *possible* to be vegan whatever your sport and at whatever level you play or compete, athletes of all calibres are increasingly saying eating plant-based has *improved* their training and performance in a number of ways. Among the most common findings are that being vegan reduces inflammation and muscle fatigue, lessens recovery time, reduces body fat, and allows athletes to train harder and stronger, all with no loss of muscle mass or strength. No wonder, topflight athletes across all disciplines are making the change.

VEGAN ATHLETES

Formula One driver Lewis Hamilton is vegan, as is former heavyweight boxer David Haye. World champion tennis player Novak Djokovic is so taken with plant-based foods that he opened his own vegan restaurant, while tennis champions Serena and Venus Williams also tout the benefits of eating plant-based while in training.

If you think eating vegan will make you weak, think again. Patrik Baboumian is an Iranian-born German retired strongman – once Germany's Strongest Man, in fact – who has set four world records in various strength disciplines and could bench-press 463lb and deadlift 794lb. He said: 'My strength needs no victims.' The list of other powerful athletes includes Olympian weightlifter Kendrick Farris, and strength athletes Nimai Delgado, Jahina Malik, Torre Washington and Anastasia Zinchenko.

Do you like a little more contact in your sport but worry that going vegan will somehow make you soft? Look at the careers of mixed martial arts champion Mac Danzig, European jiu-jitsu champion Emilia Tuukkanen or Austrian champion boxer Melanie Fraunschiel. All 100 per cent vegan, all 100 per cent badass.

'Rugby is a high-collision contact sport so no matter what you eat or what you do, you're going to be sore from the knocks and the bruises. But since going vegan I can't really remember the last time I had delayed onset muscle soreness. And that obviously helps me give more to the next training session.'
Anthony Mullally, professional rugby league player, UK

As for runners, you'd be hard-pressed to keep pace with Morgan Mitchell, Scott Jurek and Fiona Oakes. Morgan is a sprinter who represented Australia at the Olympic Games. Scott won the Western States 100-mile endurance race no fewer than seven times and has set ten ultramarathon records. Fiona, an amateur marathon runner who holds three world records, has come in the top 10 in several international marathons and in the top 20 in both London and Berlin. Oh, and remember Carl Lewis? Yep – he was vegan too.

'Being vegan has helped me immensely. I don't feel sluggish like I did when I was eating meat, and my recovery from training really took off. It felt like an overall cleanse for my body, and I started seeing greater results on the track.'

Morgan Mitchell, Olympic sprinter, Australia

Rugby league international Anthony Mullally and FIFA Women's World Cup champ Alex Morgan are vegan, and so are a whole host of NFL players including Griff Whalen, Cam Newton and Colin Kaepernick. World Champion figure skater Meagan Duhamel, cyclist Johanna Jahnke and champion surfer Tia Blanco are all vegan, too, showing that no matter what your sport, you can thrive, take titles and smash records on a vegan diet.

WHAT SHOULD A VEGAN ATHLETE EAT?

That very much depends on your sport, what you are hoping to achieve, the kinds of foods you already eat, and your own tastes and preferences. Obviously, the basic nutrition principles will always apply, but if you do sport of any kind you'll find it even easier to exceed all your micronutrient requirements simply because you are able to eat more.

Most professional athletes stick to a very specific nutrition regime that is difficult for amateurs to emulate but in truth every athlete eats differently. Some increase the amount of whole grains in their diet, others ramp up the protein. Some count calories, others keep a close eye on their carbs-protein-fat ratios. What we would say is that, where your training allows, it is good to experiment a little. The received wisdom is often wrong, and even where it is right, it is unlikely to be right for everyone. Where the layperson may think they need to eat more protein, endurance athletes often report that it was a reduction in protein that improved their performance. Be open-minded, experiment and find what works for you.

That said, most vegan athletes favour the wholefood approach and may start the day with oatmeal, smoothies, or frozen bananas made into an ice cream – all with added chia seeds, flax, fruits, seeds and nuts for healthy fats, vitamins, minerals and protein. Tia Blanco recommends adding a spoonful of molasses to breakfast each day to increase iron and calcium.

For lunch, food bowls that include quinoa, kale, nuts, olives, raw veggies, sweet potato, hummus, beans, seaweed and avocado often hit the spot. As an evening meal, athletes may choose a stir-fry with broccoli and tofu or tempeh, spinach lasagne, dahl, black bean burgers, mac n cashew cheese, or chilli made with soya mince or lentils.

Those who need a high-calorie intake may increase avocados and nuts, while adding in vegan sausages or burgers. Those requiring a big protein hike may choose vegan powders and incorporate them into smoothies, flapjacks or oatmeal.

Veganuary has created a Sports Nutrition Meal Plan with links to a week's worth of recipes that can help you achieve optimal nutrition – simply download it from the website.

To find out more about how eating vegan can be just the boost your athletic performance needs, we recommend watching *The Game Changers* movie.

VEGAN WITH ALLERGIES

While being vegan when you have food allergies can be challenging, it is not impossible, and how easy it will be very much depends on the allergy! Obviously a dairy or shellfish allergy poses no additional problem as vegans don't eat those anyway, but if you are allergic to nuts, soya or gluten, there is bound to be more to consider, and it may take a little longer to transition to a fully vegan diet.

The good news is that there is a burgeoning market in vegan free-from foods, and every supermarket in the UK now carries a wide range. Veganuary has also produced weekly meal plans for those with gluten, nut and soya allergies, with links to recipes for breakfast, lunch, dinner and a snack. They are available freely at veganuary.com, and there are many dedicated websites, blogs and recipe books to help those with allergies who wish to be vegan.

THE GLUTEN-FREE VEGAN

Gluten is the protein found in wheat, and those with coeliac disease or an allergy to gluten need to find alternatives to many common wheat-based products including bread, pasta, cakes and sauces. Thankfully, there are gluten-free vegan versions available for all these products.

Where things may get tricky is with certain meat-style vegan products such as 'bacon' or 'chicken nuggets' which are sometimes made with seitan. This is a wheat protein and so gluten-free vegans should opt instead for similar products that are made with soya or pea protein. If your local store does not stock them, search online and you'll almost certainly find what you are looking for.

There are also some very tasty gluten-free recipes on the Veganuary website – including butternut squash and sage lasagne, mushroom and thyme risotto, and blueberry pancakes – and thousands more available online. There are also several fantastic cookbooks that are dedicated to gluten-free vegan cooking, so whether you love to cook or prefer to rely on convenience foods – or a bit of both – being gluten-free does not have to stop you from becoming vegan, too.

When it comes to eating out, restaurants are increasingly learning to adapt to their customers' needs. Most pizza restaurants offer a gluten-free base and vegan cheese, so you just need to pick the toppings. And other chain and independent restaurants will almost certainly have something available, too. There is no denying that being both gluten-free and vegan is likely to limit your choices when eating out, so it is best to do your research so you go to a place where you know you will get a meal that you'll like.

THE NUT-FREE VEGAN

Nut allergies can be extremely serious, and those who are at risk will already know exactly what foods they can and can't eat, and whether they feel safe eating out.

For those with nut allergies who wish to become vegan, there are a few things to watch out for. Obviously, peanut butter is a much-loved vegan staple and can find its way into a surprising number of dishes, including sauces, cakes and pancakes. If you're cooking at home, you can substitute a nut-free version, or even use Biscoff spread.

When it comes to plant milk, choose oat, soya or rice milk over cashew or almond, and most commercially available vegan cheeses are based either on soya or coconut, but check the label to be sure as some are made with cashews.

Nuts provide good fats, protein, vitamin E, iron, zinc and magnesium. Brazil nuts are also a great source of selenium. It isn't difficult to get these nutrients as a vegan, so if you don't eat nuts, instead try seeds like chia, flax, pumpkin, sunflower and sesame.

For inspiration and some tasty nut-free recipes, visit the Veganuary website and download the Nut-Free Meal Plan.

Online, you'll also find some excellent blogs and recipe sites specifically for nut-free vegans.

THE SOYA-FREE VEGAN

Once upon a time, almost every vegan food seemed to be based around soya, but this is certainly no longer the case. There are now many more milks readily available, including rice, hemp, oat, cashew and almond, while dairy-free cheeses are often based on cashews or coconut. Similarly, there are soya-free yoghurts, ice cream and cream so there is no need to miss out on any of life's luxuries.

Some of the vegan meats you'll find have soya as their base, but many others are made from wheat or pea protein, so you'll need to read a few labels before you find the ones that are right for you. And of course, although tofu and tempeh are out, seitan (wheat protein) is very much in! Although we tend to associate soya with protein, it's not the only vegan source by a long stretch, and gram for gram seitan packs a more powerful protein punch. And of course, you can boost protein further with lentils, beans, chickpeas, nuts and seeds.

Soya products are often fortified with – or in the case of tofu, set with – calcium, so if you don't eat soya, you'll need to make sure you get sufficient from other foods. You can switch to fortified rice or oat milks and yoghurts, and add in plenty of pulses, green leafy vegetables, sesame seeds and tahini, dried fruit and bread (in many countries, including the UK, white and brown flours are fortified with calcium and other nutrients by law).

For at-home meals, check out Veganuary's Soya-free Meal Plan which offers many tasty options including black bean chilli, no-chicken coronation sandwich and Moroccan lentil, chickpea and kale soup. You can download the meal plan for free from the website.

And as for eating out, most restaurants now offer a good range of innovative plant-based meals, and very few rely on tofu as the vegan option. Pizza restaurants often use rice as the basis of their dairy-free mozzarella, making them a good choice. But most places that cater for vegans will have soya-free options on the menu. Asian restaurants may use soya in a number of their dishes, so check their allergen information online or make a phone call before you go.

VEGAN MYTHS

There are a lot of myths surrounding veganism and you're likely to be faced with at least one of them during your first few weeks as a vegan. Some myths, like, *'You won't get enough protein'*, are so common that we can pretty much predict them. Here are the most likely, and all the information you'll need to bat them away. Politely, of course.

1. What's the point? One person won't make a difference

Au contraire. One person makes a very real difference!

The average British meat-eater consumes more than 11,000 animals in their lifetime,[1] and many more animals are killed in the dairy and egg industries. By choosing to stop eating these products today, *a lot* of lives will be spared. It won't save the animals who are in farms and slaughterhouses right now, of course, but it is a simple rule of economics that when demand decreases, so does supply. As people buy fewer animal products, supermarkets and butchers reduce their orders, and fewer animals are bred and killed. A growing number of farmers are already changing from farming animals to growing crops, fruits and vegetables, and this trend will only continue.

Not only are we sparing the lives of animals when we become vegan, we're shrinking our food-related carbon emissions by up to 73 per cent.[2] Climate change is the biggest threat to people and the planet right now, and everything each of us can do to reduce our own impact is meaningful.

What we achieve alone, then, is significant but our impact is magnified so much further because we are not going vegan all by ourselves. Think of it like this: when we drop a coin into a charity box, we don't assume our pound has saved the day. No, we understand that our contribution is important but it's when lots of people also drop a pound in the box that big change comes.

And big change is already happening! There are millions of us choosing to eat only animal-free foods and each of us influences others to enjoy plant-based meals, too. In fact, more than half of the people who take part in Veganuary say they have inspired someone else to go vegan. If those people influence someone else too . . . well, you see how this works? We don't always know the impact we'll have but just by being a vegan out in the world, we normalise it and inspire others to make changes, too.

Together, the millions-strong vegan community is dramatically reducing animal suffering and climate chaos. We are also reducing the likelihood of antibiotic resistance since worldwide, 66 per cent of all antibiotics are used in farmed animals,[3] And, since three-quarters of all emerging infectious diseases begin in animals,[4] we are protecting people world-wide by reducing the risk of future pandemics, too.

What we achieve alone is something extraordinary to be proud of. Collectively, our actions are changing the whole world for the better, and every person's contribution counts.

2. Animals on high-welfare farms have a good life and a humane death

The majority of farmed animals are reared intensively. If the package on the shelf doesn't specifically say 'free range' or 'organic' then the animal was almost certainly factory-farmed, and there is no point trying to kid ourselves that those chicken nuggets came from birds who spent their days roaming free. Even where we do make the effort to choose higher-welfare meat, the reality for those animals may be very different to what we imagine. We may think of free-range hens roaming in a pasture, pigs grubbing in a woodland or goats running around an expansive hillside. In most cases, this comforting vision is a very long way from reality.

Free-range hens do not live outdoors but instead are given access to it for a period of the day, if the weather permits. Since flock sizes are enormous and hens are territorial, many birds won't cross another's territory to get to the exit holes and they'll instead spend their entire lives inside a shed. And what of the outdoor space itself? Often, it's little more than a patch of dirt, and almost certainly not what is printed on the box, shown on the website, or the image you have in your mind.

Male chicks born into the free-range egg industry will be gassed, crushed or minced alive on their first day of life because they are deemed useless. And when the females' productivity declines, being free range or organic won't save them from the slaughterhouse.

The vast majority of chickens reared for their meat are kept inside factory farms, but those who are reared under 'high-welfare' schemes fare little better. For many, the painful joint problems that are endemic in the modern high-yielding breeds mean their lives are miserable no matter what system they are reared in. When they are just a few weeks old, they are caught by their legs or necks, rammed into crates and trucked to the slaughterhouse.

For other animals, like pigs, free range usually means a patch of dirt and a metal arc. Pigs love to root, run and play. They like to socialise, build nests and explore; but none of this is afforded them on most commercial 'high-welfare' farms.

There is no humane way to produce commercial quantities of milk. Cows, goats and sheep are repeatedly made pregnant with their offspring often no more than unwanted by-products. Calves may go for veal production or be shot at birth. Cows who have their young taken away can bellow for them for days.

In some countries, cows are able to live outdoors all year round but in most parts of the world, even under 'high-welfare' schemes, they are permitted out for just six months a year. So, rather than making them stand out in the mud as the rain lashes down for the other half of the year, they are forced to stand around in their own faeces inside a barn. It's not clear which is preferable.

All animals – whether free range, organic, barn-reared, outdoor-bred or caged – end their lives in the same place. Investigations all around the world show that animals are terrified when they enter the slaughterhouse, and that those who were reared under 'high-welfare' schemes are treated no better than those reared on factory farms.

3. Why are vegans so preachy?

It's easy to think that all vegans are preachy because we tend to remember the ones who are! But of course you will have met dozens of other vegans – at work, at the gym, through your everyday life – without knowing they were vegan simply because they didn't mention it. We know that going on about our food choices can make some people uncomfortable, even angry, but nonetheless we are going to mount a defence of preachy vegans. Bear with us.

Have you seen the film *The Matrix*? Of course you have. And remember the question at its very heart: Do you want to know the truth, difficult as it may be, or would you rather live in comfortable ignorance, plugged into the matrix? New vegans often feel as though they have just unplugged themselves and are seeing the world for the very first time. They see how illogical it is to eat pigs but adopt a rescued dog, and that being concerned about the climate crisis matters little if we ignore the 'single biggest way'[5] we can reduce our own impact on the planet. They see the devastation caused by animal agriculture on the world's forests, wildlife, rivers, streams and oceans. They see how our diet is behind some of the leading causes of death in the western world, and that by eating plant-based, people can reduce their risks. They see for the very first time that meat, eggs and dairy are not somehow part of the fabric of life, but that these are things we can simply choose not to eat. And, without wishing to be dramatic, it is a complete and utter revelation! To use another film analogy, it's like the curtain is drawn back but there is no wonderful wizard sitting there, just a global marketing strategy trying to get us to eat a product that causes all this damage. In that moment, they realise they have been hoodwinked all their lives, so it's no wonder new vegans can get a little exuberant.

So, we'd urge you to focus on the message, not the messenger. After all, vegans are just trying to make the world a better place. Annoying as that may be.

4. It's natural to eat meat

What is 'natural'? The chicken who cannot live more than six weeks, the turkey who can't even breed without human help or the cow selectively bred to produce far more milk than is good for her health?

Farmed animals are artificially inseminated, endure many mutilations and are selectively bred to have large litters. They're engineered to put on weight fast, unless they're a hen farmed for eggs or a cow used for dairy production, in which case they're bred *not* to put on weight, as that would be a waste of food. They are fed artificial feed, have their breeding cycles manipulated with hormone sponges inserted into their vaginas[6] and the length of their day is managed through artificial lighting. It's not possible to imagine anything less natural than the animal farming industry.

Often what people mean by this is, *Haven't we always done it?* and *Don't we have all the right biological equipment to eat meat?* And the answers to those questions are *no* and *not really.*

The food our ancestors ate would have depended on what era they lived in and where in the world, as well as the season, the climate and the weather, so we can't make any generalisations about what we have 'always eaten'.

We do know that early humans were predominantly gatherers like other apes, only scavenging meat that true carnivores left behind. Take a look at our hands and teeth, which are useless for ripping flesh, and our lack of speed, which would see even a lame antelope outrun us. These things are not a problem for true carnivores, like jaguars and tigers. The canine teeth people cite as 'proof' that we should eat meat look nothing like the canines of carnivores and are misnamed.

Obviously, we can tolerate a bit of meat in our diet, but our bodies have never really adapted to significant quantities of it. Our intestines are long, and look more like those belonging to our herbivorous friends than to our carnivorous ones. Carnivores have short intestines as they need to move meat out of their system quickly before it putrefies and kills them. Food poisoning in people is still predominantly caused by animal products and meat continues to harm the human body in many other ways, including through higher rates of heart disease, some cancers and diabetes.

5. You'll feel weak or ill

Vegan food is nutritious and the vast majority of people who take part in Veganuary say they feel better as a result of going without animal products. Even within the first few weeks, many report that they have more energy, have lost weight and sleep better. Many also say they have improved digestion, skin, hair and nails.

For most people, switching to a vegan diet feels great in the short term, but crucially it also reduces their risks over the long term from diseases like cancer, heart disease and diabetes.

If someone becomes ill when they switch to a vegan diet, then generally one of two things is happening: either they have caught a bug or developed a condition and would have become ill anyway, or they are eating all the wrong foods.

With so many convenience foods available, it's entirely possible to be a junk food vegan and if you fail to eat good, wholesome, nutritious foods, it's obvious you're more likely to feel under the weather. That's true whatever your diet. If a person chooses to live off biscuits and crisps, you can't really blame their deficiencies on veganism. It's their food choices that are the problem. Conversely, if they eat a balanced diet then they're very unlikely to become ill as a result.

All the nutrients you need can be found in a well-planned vegan diet. So if you find you're falling short of, say, iron, then make sure you include plenty of whole grains, beans, peas, nut butters and green leafy vegetables in your diet.

Online nutrition trackers and apps can be useful in giving you a rough idea about whether you are consistently failing to get enough of a particular nutrient. If this is the case, you'll need to adjust your diet to account for it, but the good news is that this can all be done on a vegan diet, and there's no need to go back to the animal products that can cause so much sickness in the long run.

It may take a little time to adapt and get into the groove of a vegan diet, and you may notice some changes to your body in that time – including in your weight, skin and frequency of bathroom visits – but if you start to experience unpleasant symptoms, don't make assumptions about the cause. Instead see a doctor for advice. And remember it takes a little time for a good diet to undo the damage of a poor one.

6. What will farmers do if everyone goes vegan?

Farmers grow all our foods: the wheat and other grains we have in our bread and pasta, the fruits, herbs, salads, legumes, nuts, spices and other vegetables. They grow all the ingredients in our vegan cheese, plant milk, our nuggets, pies, burgers and other foods. Farmers will keep growing these products and we will keep buying and eating them.

Farmers have always adapted to changing markets. They are used to changing what they grow to take advantage of farm subsidies and they have always adapted to consumer preferences. Already, many farmers can see the way the world is changing and are moving away from rearing animals in favour of growing crops. Besides, we can't keep buying meat just to keep one aspect of an industry going. If we did that, we'd still be buying coal when we could be buying clean energy, or disposable coffee cups when we could instead drink from a reusable one. Farming is like any industry – it will thrive because we want to buy its products, but it cannot tell us what products we should choose. Imagine a supermarket welcoming you in and then berating you for choosing one product over another!

And don't worry about there being fewer jobs in farming. Horticulture – the growing of fruits, vegetables and flowers – is the most labour-intensive of all the different agricultural sub-sectors, so the more plants we eat, the more jobs there are.

7. Veganism is too expensive

An independent study commissioned by Veganuary in 2020 found that, on average, plant-based meals eaten at home cost 40 per cent less than meat or fish-based meals. The research was conducted by Kantar which records online weekly meal diaries from around 11,000 people in Britain. By analysing these, it found that a main meal containing meat, fish or poultry costs, on average, £1.77 per person whereas a plant-based main meal costs just £1.06 per person. This is a saving of 71p per person per meal.

Kantar also continuously tracks purchases from 30,000 British households and found that vegan households spend 8 per cent less per grocery trip, on average, than non-vegan households of a similar size. Perhaps it's not that surprising when you consider just how expensive a piece of meat or fish is.

It's true that most plant-based milk and cheese is pricier than most of their dairy equivalents, but overall the cost of the weekly shop is likely to come down, as we load up with seasonal vegetables and plenty of wholegrains, and leave those costly pieces of meat on the shelves.

You should notice the same when you eat out. The most expensive items on the menu tend to be meat-based while the cheapest ones are plant-based. And the reason is simple: chickpeas are cheaper than chicken, and beans are cheaper than beef.

8. We have canine teeth so . . .

Have you seen a tiger's canine teeth? They look nothing like ours! And that's because theirs are used for puncturing, holding and ripping flesh whereas ours are really only useful for biting through carrots. We need to accept that someone, somewhere has mislabelled these teeth. They certainly do not indicate that we are 'natural meat-eaters'.

There are other clues in our body as well. Look at the claws you possess. They are powerful and razor-sharp and can rip apart an animal in seconds. No? That's because our hands are mobile and dexterous, perfect for picking fruits, and the nails we have protect the delicate ends of our fingers. There is not a talon in sight.

Next we should consider our guts. If we could pull them out, they would stretch to around 20 feet long which is why it takes up to 48 hours for food to transit through the colon. The intestines of a true carnivore are shorter than ours, because they need to get the meat in, digested and back out of their systems before it putrefies.

And what about the bloodlust we all feel every day? Again, no? Most of us do not have the motivation to go out and kill. It's just not in our natures. And even if we had the motivation, could we actually outrun a wild animal and bring him or her down?

Now, you might counter: but we have evolved to let others do all that for us. And we might counter your counter and say: so we've turned our backs on all that is considered natural and yet we are still happy to cite this one tooth as proof that we should naturally eat meat. We might as well say the coccyx is proof that we really should be swinging from trees.

And so we might bat the argument back and forth all day but the bottom line is this: obviously, like other apes we can tolerate some meat in our diets but evidence overwhelmingly shows that our bodies thank us when we fuel them with plants. Vegans suffer less from heart disease, obesity, type 2 diabetes and there is some evidence they live longer, too.

9. Isn't soya destroying our planet?

Large expanses of land are needed to grow the quantity of soya beans the world requires, and swathes of ancient forests and savannah have been felled as a result.[7] Deforestation is devastating for biodiversity and these ancient ecosystems, once felled, are lost for ever.

It's easy to blame the people who eat tofu or drink soya milk because they're the most visible consumers of these beans. But they are not the *main* consumers of soya. Most of the world's crop, in fact, is fed to farmed animals,[8] including to fish.[9] Most of the world's soya is eaten by meat-eaters, albeit indirectly.

We have to acknowledge that all farming has an impact on the environment, and that the land we use to grow any food may be less diverse and sustain fewer species than had it been left in a wild state. But the advice given by the World

Wild Fund for Nature for reducing the amount of soya grown is to limit consumption of animal products and, in particular, meat.[10]

Vegans who have an allergy to soya find it's perfectly possible to get sufficient protein from other plant sources, so it is not essential that a plant-based diet include this bean. But soya itself isn't the problem. Trying to grow enough soya to feed billions of farmed animals is.

10. The 'desert island' myth

This is less of a myth and more of a question: *If you were stranded on a desert island, would you eat meat then?*

We need to be straight with you. You're no more likely to be stranded on a desert island after going vegan than you were before, but you will be asked about it so often that there may be times when you wish you were stranded far, far away.

Since there is unlikely to be a delicatessen on this island, the question isn't so much *Would you eat meat?* as *Would you kill an animal?* We can overlook for now how these animals came to be on the island, and we could answer simply that, however they got there, they appear to be thriving, so we'll just eat what they're eating. It is a lot safer to eat nuts, roots, tubers and berries than to hunt down wild beasts with a stick. (We're assuming we didn't get washed up with a loaded gun, a set of butchery knives, *Evisceration for Dummies* and a camping stove.)

Animals don't walk over and lie down for you, you know. You'd have to track them, surprise them, overpower them and cut their throats. In this struggle, there's a decent chance that you'll be the one who ends up as someone's dinner. No offence. It's just that they're a wild animal and have spent their whole life successfully not getting eaten and you're, you know, an accountant or a teacher or a bus driver.

The savvy will have spotted that this question is not really about desert islands, it's about finding the limit to your resolve and principles. *Would you really rather starve to death than eat an animal?* This question can be flipped on the questioner: *If you were living on an island with loads of wholesome plant-based foods, would you still choose to eat the corpses of tortured animals?*

Failing that approach, you can usually stop the conversation with: *If I was hungry enough, I would eat you.*

MEAL PLANS

If you don't quite know where to start, we've created a series of meal plans to help you, and they can all be found at veganuary.com. They include a 'quick and convenient' plan, a family-friendly plan, as well as plans for athletes, those who love to cook, and those avoiding gluten, soya and nuts.

'Definitely do it. There's no downside to signing up for Veganuary. You can participate to the extent that you want – just read and ponder the daily emails, which contain recipes, info about some of the issues and inspiring stories; or go ahead and try some of the recipes; or decide to have 'meat-free Monday' each week; or dive in and commit to eating no animal products at all for the month.'

Heather K., Victoria, Australia,
Veganuary Class of 2017

Below are two meal plans for fledgling vegans. The first is for your very first week transitioning to a vegan diet, and contains simple favourites to get you started. The second is for when you're feeling a bit more adventurous and you're ready to test your vegan wings. You'll find the <u>underlined</u> recipes at veganuary.com/recipes.

MEAL PLAN 1

Getting Started: Keeping it simple

Monday

BREAKFAST

<u>Porridge/oatmeal with bananas and seeds</u>, made with a plant milk of your choice – remember some come sweetened, some don't.

LUNCH

Falafel, rocket (arugula) and sweet chilli sauce sandwich

DINNER

<u>Shepherd's pie</u>, using soya mince or lentils instead of meat. Remember dairy-free butter and milk for the mashed potato!

Tuesday

BREAKFAST

Breakfast cereal of your choice with dairy-free yoghurt

LUNCH

<u>Vegetable soup</u> (either bought or home-made using vegetable stock) with crusty bread

DINNER

Fajitas. Use vegan meat strips or strips of seitan or tofu, or try these <u>portobello fajitas</u>. Serve with guacamole and salsa

Wednesday

BREAKFAST

Avocado and tomatoes on toast

LUNCH

<u>Quinoa Mexicana salad</u>, made with avocado, kidney beans, chilli and lime

DINNER

<u>Pasta arrabbiata</u> (or keep it simple and buy a jar of pasta sauce), served with a green salad and garlic bread

Thursday

BREAKFAST

Fruit smoothie and wholemeal toast with your choice
of peanut butter, yeast extract or jam

LUNCH

Veggie sausage sandwich with mustard or ketchup,
some salad leaves and tomatoes

DINNER

Courgette and sun-dried tomato risotto. Serve with
asparagus, broccoli or a mixed salad

Friday

BREAKFAST

Super-healthy, superfood yoghurt – your choice of
dairy-free yoghurt with berries, fruit, nuts and seeds

LUNCH

Hummus and salad wraps – choose your flavour of
hummus and your favourite veg

DINNER

Pizza – either a shop-bought vegan pizza or buy the
dough base and add tomato sauce, your choice of
toppings and dairy-free cheese

Saturday

BREAKFAST

Maple cinnamon granola (make this the day before)

LUNCH

Roasted red pepper soup with cheese on toast

DINNER

Bangers and mash. Your choice of vegan sausages, with mashed potatoes, peas and vegan gravy

Sunday

BREAKFAST

The full fried breakfast: choose from vegan sausages and bacon, tofu scramble, grilled tomatoes, fried mushrooms, baked beans and toast or 'veggy' bread

LUNCH

Ginger, coconut and lemongrass soup

DINNER

Roast dinner. All your favourite roast potatoes, parsnips, carrots and celeriac with a centrepiece of your choice. Why not try 'chicken' and leek pie, mushroom and chestnut wellington or herby stuffed squash?

MEAL PLAN 2

Going Gourmet: OK, let's do this vegan thing

Monday

BREAKFAST

Psychedelic smoothie bowl – a bright, nutrient-rich breakfast bowl

LUNCH

Speedy sweet potato quesadillas with salad

DINNER

Vegan butter chicken with rice or quinoa

Tuesday

BREAKFAST

Choc and raspberry porridge

LUNCH

Vegan quiche served with a Waldorf salad

DINNER

Beetroot and kale burgers with balsamic red onions

Wednesday

BREAKFAST

Banana pancakes with blueberries and maple syrup

LUNCH

Portobello mushrooms and tofu scramble ciabatta sandwich

DINNER

Black bean chilli with rice and a green salad

Thursday

BREAKFAST

Apple cinnamon wholemeal waffles (waffle maker needed)

LUNCH

Chilli tomato and basil baked beans on toast

DINNER

Mixed root vegetable gnocchi in sage-pistachio pesto

Friday

BREAKFAST

Breakfast burritos

LUNCH

Carrot and coriander soup with sourdough chilli croutons

DINNER

BBQ pulled jackfruit with corn tacos

Saturday

BREAKFAST

Toast with garlicky butterbean toast topper

LUNCH

Warm potato salad with chargrilled asparagus and lemon

DINNER

Turkish tofu and spinach börek

Sunday

BREAKFAST

Tortilla Española

LUNCH

Leek latkes with cauliflower cheese

DINNER

Roasted vegetable lasagne

SNACKS:

Fresh fruit, dried fruit, crackers with vegan cheese, crisps, dairy-free chocolate, cereal bars and mixed nuts. For the weekend, why not make <u>espresso doughnuts, peach Danish pastries, cookies, spiced plum muffins or brownies</u>?

DRINKS:

Fruit juice, coffee, tea, herbal tea, water, squash – whatever you normally have

DESSERTS:

Choose from the many delicious desserts at veganuary.com, including our favourites: <u>lemon tarts, banoffee pie, pomegranate cheesecake</u> and <u>nutty chocolate truffles</u>. There are some healthier options, too!

FOUR MIND-BLOWING RECIPES THAT GIVE AWAY VEGAN SECRETS!

'I'd tried to be a vegetarian a number of times over the years but always slipped back. I guess with Veganuary I thought that, at best, I'd learn a few recipes to add to weekly meals. I never imagined that over the course of the month I'd take on a full vegan diet!'

Melanie R., Lennoxtown, Scotland,
Veganuary Class of 2017

This is not a recipe book but we did want to share with you four of our favourite recipes to let you in on some of the best-kept secrets of the vegan world: aquafaba, flaxseed, nooch and jackfruit. Prepare to be amazed.

Meringues

(SERVES 6)

There is magic in the world. And if you don't believe us try this egg-free meringue recipe, made using the brine from a can of chickpeas. Sounds gross, we know, but when whipped, sweetened and baked you absolutely cannot tell it apart from traditional meringues. For a beautifully gentle floral flavour, add some rosewater or make them without if you prefer. You'll need an electric whisk and some patience but these are oh so worth the wait.

INGREDIENTS

100ml aquafaba (either bought in a carton, or retrieved and sieved from a can of chickpeas)
¼ tsp cream of tartar
100g caster sugar
½ tsp vanilla extract
½ tsp rosewater (optional)

INSTRUCTIONS

- Put a large mixing bowl into the freezer to cool for 20 minutes.
- Heat the oven to 100C.
- Cover a baking tray in greaseproof paper and set aside.
- Beat the aquafaba and cream of tartar on high speed until soft peaks form – around 8-10 minutes.

- Add the sugar one tablespoon at a time and beat, again on high speed until stiff peaks form – around another 10 minutes.
- Add the vanilla essence and rosewater (if using), and beat for another minute.
- Drop tablespoon-sized blobs of the mixture onto the greaseproof paper and bake in the oven for 1 hour, 45 minutes until they are fairly firm on the top and base. Switch off the oven, open the door and let them remain in the oven until cool.

To make a pavlova, follow this recipe and make six disc-shaped meringues instead of mini meringues. When cool, top with whippable vegan cream (available in many supermarkets and health food shops) and strawberries.

Crepes

(MAKES 8 PANCAKES)

Those wafer-thin soft and delicious pancakes that are a dream with sugar and lemon, drizzled with syrup, or made savoury and stuffed with anything you like. Surely those need eggs in them? Nope. The secret here is ground flaxseed which, when combined with a little water, does the job of the egg in this and many other recipes. Try it!

INGREDIENTS

1 tbsp ground flax
125g plain flour
300ml plant milk
1 tbsp caster sugar
¼ tsp salt
sunflower oil

INSTRUCTIONS

- Combine the flaxseed with 3 tbsp of warm water and set aside until it has a jelly-like consistency (just a minute or two).
- Sift the flour, stir in the milk, then the flaxseed, sugar and salt.
- Heat a little oil in a non-stick frying pan over a medium heat. When hot, add half a ladle of the mixture, swirling it round to coat the base of the pan. You want the pancake as thin as possible.
- Cook for 2 minutes, then flip and cook for one more.

Queso (cheese dip)
(MAKES ONE BOWL FOR SHARING)

If there is one ingredient that vegans will lose their minds over it's nutritional yeast, also known as *nooch*. It's a flaky substance that is a little bit cheesy, a little bit nutty and is often fortified with B vitamins making it a handy and nutritious accompaniment for pasta dishes, soups, stews and to sprinkle onto scrambled tofu for breakfast. This rich and cheesy dip recipe is absolutely, definitely one to try.

INGREDIENTS

150g cashews
100g red pepper
4 tbsp nutritional yeast
½ tsp garlic powder
½ tsp turmeric
½ tsp onion powder
½ tsp smoked paprika
½ tsp salt
50–100 ml stock

INSTRUCTIONS

- If your blender is not super-high power, you'll want to soak your cashews in hot water for 30 minutes, then drain.
- Then, put all the ingredients in the blender and blitz 'til smooth, adding as much stock as you need to get the consistency you like.

BBQ Pulled Jackfruit Sandwich with Slaw

(MAKES 2)

Jackfruit is a fruit that pulls apart like shredded meats, and soaks up the flavours you cook it with. It teams brilliantly with barbecue spices and while this flavour-packed sandwich never fails to please, it really couldn't be simpler to make.

It's a very handy mid-week meal when time is short, and is a winner with kids if you just dial down the heat.

INGREDIENTS
400g can jackfruit in water
3 tsp BBQ seasoning
2 tbsp olive oil, divided
75g BBQ sauce

2 buns of your choice

For the slaw:
50g celeriac, peeled
½ apple, cored
35g red cabbage
squeeze of lemon juice
3 good tbsp vegan mayo
1 tsp Dijon mustard
handful parsley, chopped

INSTRUCTIONS
- Drain and rinse the jackfruit, then cut out the fruit's hard core and shred the rest with your fingers.
- Mix well with the BBQ seasoning and 1 tbsp oil, and set aside for at least 30 minutes.
- Meanwhile, make the slaw by grating or shredding finely the celeriac, apple and red cabbage. Then mix in the lemon juice, mayo, mustard and parsley.

- Heat a non-stick frying pan and cook the jackfruit in 1 tbsp oil over a medium heat until for about 5 minutes.
- Add the BBQ sauce and cook for another 3-4 minutes.
- Serve in a bun, topped with the slaw.

THE BIG QUESTIONS

For new vegans and those just dipping their toes into the plant-based pool, there are inevitably a lot of questions that crop up. The Veganuary website and our social media platforms are great places to start searching for additional advice and information, but there are a few questions that may still linger in your mind, and not everyone feels able to voice these aloud. We hear you, and we hope this section helps.

WHAT IF I MESS UP?

So, you've pledged to try vegan for 31 days. You're armed with as much info as your head can hold and you've read every label in the supermarket. Your cupboards are packed with plant-based foods and you've calculated how many steps lie between you and your nearest vegan burrito. You've registered to take part in Veganuary, which you can do at any time of year if you don't want to wait until January, and those support emails will be arriving in your inbox any moment. You are on your vegan way. But still you worry, *What if I mess up?*

There is no messing up. Taking part in Veganuary signals that you're going to give plant-based eating a good go for those 31 days, but there is no one hiding in your fridge to leap out at you if you come home with a cheese-crusted pizza late one night. You won't be shamed on social media or outed on the national news.

If you make a mistake or have a slip-up, it's OK. These things happen, and we've been there. Old habits don't always let go of us, even if we're trying our hardest to shake them off. And even the best-intentioned resolve can weaken after a drink or two. Our advice is: don't let it set you back. If you really want to stick with trying vegan, put the lapse to the back of your mind. You just made a mistake, so start again tomorrow.

'I just wanted to say that this has been the most supportive group I have ever joined! I have enjoyed Veganuary, one or two slip-ups, but I am learning to forgive myself. I have loved the way we have shared and discussed options.'

Rachel J., Stockport, UK, Veganuary Class of 2017

I'M STRUGGLING! WHAT SHOULD I DO?

No one is underestimating how challenging it is to change lifelong food habits, especially when those around you are continuing to eat what they've always eaten. Nights out, meals with friends and special occasions can all take some getting used to, and for some people, trying vegan can feel like a lonely experience. And on those days when all you can think about is your cravings for cheese, it's hard to remember why you ever thought trying vegan was a good idea. If you know deep down that you'd like to try or be vegan but you're struggling to stick with it, these top tips might just get you through.

- Remind yourself why you're doing this! Write down all the reasons why you wanted to give veganism a try, and see if they remain. Re-read the *Why Try Vegan?* section of this book, and check out the books and films we recommend on pages 197–199.

- Connect with other vegans by joining vegan groups in real life or online. Even if you are the only vegan you know, you are not alone. There are millions of us on your side! Check out the next section for advice on finding your vegan tribe.

- Read the testimonials within this book. They're inspirational, and written by people who have experienced exactly what you're experiencing, and have got through it.

- Remember it's OK to take it slow. It may be better to replace one product at a time and transition over a period than to leap straight in if you're finding it difficult. If there's one thing you think you'll miss most of all, take the pressure off yourself and leave that until last. There are no rules about becoming vegan. Take it at a pace that works for you.

- Keep a diary so you can remind yourself how far you've come and what you've already achieved, how amazing you felt on the good days, the new favourite foods that you've discovered and why this is important to you. Writing it down can make it much more real, and help you work through any issues you may be having.

- Be good to yourself. Being vegan isn't about deprivation. Treat yourself with a bar of chocolate (not just the dark ones; there are lots of vegan 'milk' chocolates available), a glass of wine or a meal out at your favourite vegan cafe or restaurant. Try to make your vegan journey a joyful experience.

- Watch a movie. Not one of the ones that will keep you awake at night but something like Cowspiracy or Vegucated that will inspire you and strengthen your resolve. We all have days when we struggle. These films can remind us why we are taking a stand. Throw in some popcorn and everything will seem just a little bit brighter.

- If what you are learning is overwhelming you, please know that the issues around veganism are HUGE, and it's normal to be saddened or even angry at times. If you feel your mental health is suffering, and this is something you've struggled with before, is there anything you can do that you know might help? Talking to people who understand what you're going through, meditation and other relaxation techniques perhaps, and spending time in nature has been shown to be beneficial, too. Can you switch off and go for a walk, or spend a day at an animal sanctuary? If your feelings are too much to cope with, please talk to someone who can help.

- Keep doing what you love! Nothing has to change when you become vegan apart from the ingredients in your meals. You don't have to even tell people if you don't want to! And in fact, there are times when *not* talking or thinking about veganism is very welcome. So, don't give up your old friends and hobbies unless they are very much at odds with your principles and what makes you happy.

WHERE DO I FIND
MY VEGAN TRIBE?

There is a lot to be said for spending time with like-minded people, and when you become vegan it's natural to want be around people who just 'get it'. With them, you don't need to explain your food choices, justify your views or pretend to feel something you don't. Vegans are, by and large, a caring, compassionate group of people who know how to pick you up, make you laugh and give you that support when you need it most. Finding your vegan tribe can be both a comfort and a lot of fun, and it is all part of the positive change that veganism can bring into your life. But where is your tribe?

A great place to start is online. The Veganuary Facebook group is full of supportive vegans – some of them are novices and still adjusting to their new way of life, while others are vegan veterans. Don't be afraid to voice your concerns or ask for some moral support there. And there are plenty of other online groups, too. Drop by and see which ones match your own vibe.

There are also many groups where people are connected not just by veganism but by another hobby or passion as well. This could be a vegan cyclist group, vegan knitters and crocheters, vegan gardeners, vegan metalheads, vegan musicians or vegan yogis. There are groups for vegans of faith, vegans of colour, vegans within political parties and vegan environmentalists. Whatever you're into there is probably a group!

You will also find vegan groups located near to where you live and since they often have a social element, you will be able to go along and meet them in real life, too. It could be they have a monthly meal together, or perhaps they put on events such as vegan fairs and festivals. Get involved with one of these and as you jostle with hundreds or thousands of other people to reach the cupcake stall, you'll know for certain that you're not alone!

Vegan Runners is another group that meets both online and in real life. Their members are runners of all ages and abilities and with them you can talk running tech, PBs, negative splits and sports nutrition, all while being loudly supportive of one another and, of course, quietly competitive.

If you're looking to get actively involved in changing the world for the better, you will find animal protection and environmental groups that you can support, and outreach events and demonstrations that you can attend.

And finally, if you're looking for a partner who shares your views and with whom you want to share life's journey, and perhaps change the world together, check out the vegan dating sites.

WHAT HAPPENS ON DAY 32?

Some people start their month of plant-based eating intending to be fully vegan by the end. Others are surprised that the 31-day challenge that had once seemed so daunting has become a way of life so quickly. Some people take part in Veganuary every year, and enjoy each month of plant-based eating. Others, who have taken part several times already, come to decide they will remain a full-time vegan in the future. Of those who try it but don't stay vegan, most people decide to significantly reduce their consumption of animal products.

Whatever happens, happens. All we ask is that you give it your best shot for 31 days. Only when you break some of those old habits, form some new ones, learn about the issues, try the many different products available and see how your body reacts to a fully plant-based diet – only then will you know whether you will want to stay vegan.

First and foremost, we want you to *try* vegan, but you won't be surprised to learn that we'd love you to *stay* vegan, too. That choice is yours alone, but for now, throw yourself into it. Embrace the challenge. Learn some new recipes. Make some new friends. See how your body feels. Discover what other changes it brings into your life. Be open-minded and adventurous. And on day 32 you will wake up, and you'll know what to do.

I THINK I'VE GONE VEGAN . . . WHAT NOW?

Not everyone expects to become vegan at the end of the 31 days but there are hundreds of thousands of people who surprise themselves and take to veganism like a rescued factory-farmed duck to water. For many, this is just the beginning of a lifelong adventure, and they're hungry for more.

If you've attended vegan fairs and festivals, watched speakers online, seen some of those incredible vegan documentaries or read inspirational books, you may be feeling energised to do more than just be vegan. You may feel you want to learn new skills to help you share what you have learned, and will find workshops and events that will help you learn more about outreach, public speaking and effective activism. It's not all banners and shouting! Lots of people give talks and cookery demonstrations in schools, sign petitions, share videos online, or make their own films. People write blogs, create websites and launch their own YouTube channels. Some write to newspapers, or hold a vegan coffee morning to fundraise for an animal charity. Some even decide on a career change.

You may decide to put your new nutrition to the test and set yourself a sporting challenge to raise money for a cause that is close to your heart. There are lot of ways to be an ambassador for a vegan lifestyle, not least wearing the compassionate message emblazoned across your Lycra as you knock out a plant-based PB.

If cooking is your passion, maybe you'll invite friends to a vegan meal to showcase how delicious the food can be, or take cakes or cookies into work along with the recipes for those who'd like to make them at home. Maybe you'll visit the restaurants in your town and encourage them to offer a wider range of plant-based meals. Perhaps you'll have a stall selling vegan baked goods at your local market or other event.

You might like to volunteer at your local animal sanctuary or offer a home to some rescued hens. Or you may feel, as many new vegans do, a greater connection with nature, and you'll want to spend more time outdoors, watching the sun rise or listening to birdsong. Perhaps you'll be inspired to volunteer with beach cleaning or get involved with environmental groups working to protect the natural world.

If you found this book helpful, maybe you'll buy more copies of it for friends and family, or donate one to your local library. You may like to support Veganuary and help us make more vegans.

All these things and many more are possible. But maybe none of this is for you, and you'll continue your life exactly as you did before, only you won't be eating animals.

Only you will know where veganism will take you.

RECOMMENDED READING AND VIEWING

There are some amazing books and films out there that will inspire and inform you, and these are just a few of our favourites.

Books

- *Eating Animals*, by Jonathan Safran Foer: this book changes lives! 'Gripping, horrible, wonderful, breathtaking, original. A brilliant synthesis of argument, science and storytelling. One of the finest books ever written on the subject of eating animals', says *The Times Literary Supplement*

- *Why We Love Dogs, Eat Pigs and Wear Cows*, by Melanie Joy: an introduction by this vegan social psychologist author to 'carnism' – the ideology that conditions people to see some animals as food and others as friends. A powerful, fascinating book

- *How Not to Die*, by Dr Michael Greger: scientifically proven nutritional advice on how to prevent our biggest killers – heart disease, breast and prostate cancers, diabetes and more

- *Meathooked,* by Marta Zaraska: an examination of the history of meat-eating – how it began, why it's so pervasive, and what it means for our health and our planet

- *Esther the Wonder Pig*, by Steve Jenkins and Derek Walter: a wonderfully funny, inspiring story of how Esther, a 'micropig', changed the lives and perceptions of the people who adopted her

Films

- *Cowspiracy*: follow the journey of film-maker Kip Andersen as he goes on a mission to uncover the environmental impact of our food choices. Engaging and compelling

- *Earthlings*: one of the most impactful films you will see. It's a tough watch, but one that will change how you view society's use of animals. Definitely not suitable for children

- *The Game Changers:* a must-see film about protein, strength and athleticism. Executive producers were James Cameron, Arnold Schwarzenegger, Jackie Chan, Lewis Hamilton and Novak Djokovic

- *Seaspiracy*: a powerful but alarming examination of the widespread environmental destruction caused to our oceans, and the corruption at the heart of the fishing industry

- *Forks Over Knives*: this thought-provoking, life-changing film presents the case for eating plant-based foods for our health. Always a popular choice with Veganuary participants

INFORMATION AND PRACTICAL SUPPORT

Got a question that isn't answered here? Or looking for further practical help? veganuary.com has all the info you might need, as well as hundreds of tasty recipes. Follow us on social media for inspiration, information and a few laughs.

FB: @Veganuary
IG: @WeAreVeganuary
Twitter: @Veganuary
TikTok: @Veganuary
YouTube: @Veganuary

'This was the best decision of my life. I know lots of people say it, and I certainly mean it: I wish that I had been a vegan all of my life. The only regret I have about being a vegan is that I wish I'd done it sooner.'

Peter Egan, actor, UK,
Veganuary Class of 2016 and Veganuary Ambassador

FINAL THOUGHTS

When Donald Watson coined the word *vegan* in 1944, he couldn't have imagined the worldwide movement that was going to follow. For him and his band of pioneering friends, veganism was all about ending the exploitation of animals. It was then, as it is now, a social justice movement. For many vegans, speciesism sits alongside racism and sexism as one more form of discrimination. After all, aren't we all just animals trying to do the best we can on this small planet we share?

Those early vegans wouldn't have known just how much environmental devastation that animal agriculture causes, or that people would starve while grain that could have sustained them was fed to farmed animals. Perhaps they wouldn't have known all the health benefits of a plant-based diet, either.

Today, we know a lot more. And the more we know, the more reasons we find to follow their lead.

Being vegan spares the suffering of animals that most of us cannot bear even to watch. It reduces our impact on the planet and safeguards it for the future. And it protects our health against some of the most common causes of death: heart disease, stroke, diabetes and some cancers.

Thank you for thinking more carefully about your food choices, for pledging to try veganism for a month, for one day a week or for the rest of your life. Every vegan meal we eat makes a difference. Each one is an affirmation that we want a kinder, fairer and healthier world, and that we won't wait for someone else to create it.

Trying vegan for 31 days could change your life, and if you decide once the month is over that staying vegan is the right choice for you, well, Veganuary will be on hand to advise, mentor and support you should you need it. Get in touch anyway. We'd love to hear from you.

MORE ON VEGANUARY

Veganuary (pronounced vee-GAN-uary) is a UK charity with a global reach that encourages people to try vegan in January (or any time of year), and offers support and advice throughout the process. More than one million people from almost every country in the world have already officially taken part, though the real figure is likely to be ten times higher.

Most people who sign up for the month are omnivores or pescatarians (people who eat fish but no other meat), but many are vegetarians, too. Whatever your diet, wherever you're from and whatever your age or gender, all are welcome. It's totally free to take part in Veganuary, and everyone who signs up receives:

- Daily emails with shopping lists, eating-out guides, nutrition advice, recipes, meal plans and answers to common questions

- Social media support in our closed Facebook group. Here you can connect with other participants from around the world, and share your experiences

- A free celebrity e-cookbook, with delicious animal-free recipes

- News of all the latest vegan food launches and special offers from some of your favourite companies

We aim to make the month enjoyable and interesting. We encourage and support; we never judge. Around half of those surveyed enjoy taking part in Veganuary so much that they choose to stay vegan at the end of the month, and most choose to significantly reduce their consumption of animal products. Some people take part in Veganuary every year; others take part for several years before deciding to become vegan. The path you choose is up to you.

Sign up for Veganuary today at veganuary.com or by scanning the QR code below

'Thanks to this group and its awesome support and positivity, I am so proud that I not only smashed January but have continued into March without a hiccup. This is a life choice for me now . . . one I actually always wanted to make but for some reason doubted I could do . . . so I just wanted to say *Thank you.*'

Vickie D., Millswood, South Australia,
Veganuary Class of 2017

ABOUT THE AUTHOR

Kate Schuler became vegan in 1992 after the shock of discovering that cows and chickens were killed in the dairy and egg industries as well as for meat. After her first seven days as a vegan, her resolve temporarily failed and she gorged on cheese. Afterwards, when feeling sick with guilt and sick with cheese, she vowed never to eat animal products again. Since then, she has worked with more than 20 pro-vegan organisations and businesses to make the case for a plant-based world. One mark of progress is that there are now more than a dozen vegan cheeses for sale within a mile of her home. Kate lives in Sussex, UK, and shares her home with her partner Christopher and their rescued dogs and rabbits.

NOTES

Introduction

1 'Vegan trends in the US', Ipsos Retail Performance. https://www.ipsos-retailperformance.com/en/vegan-trends/

2 'Number of vegans in Great Britain from 2014 to 2019', Statista, 2021. https://www.statista.com/statistics/1062104/number-of-vegans-in-great-britain/

3 Janet Forgrieve, 'New products, growing demand fuel growth of plant-based food sales', Forbes, 10 Mar 2020. https://www.forbes.com/sites/janetforgrieve/2020/03/10/new-products-growing-demand-fuel-growth-of-plant-based-food-sales/

4 Rebecca Smithers, 'The UK demand for new vegan food products soars in lockdown', the *Guardian*, 25 Jul 2020. https://www.theguardian.com/lifeandstyle/2020/jul/25/uk-demand-for-new-vegan-food-products-soars-in-lockdown

Why Try Vegan?

1 Lund University, 'The four lifestyle choices that most reduce your carbon footprint', 12 July 2017. https://www.lunduniversity.lu.se/article/four-lifestyle-choices-most-reduce-your-carbon-footprint

Notes

2   Hannah Ritchie and Max Roser, 'Meat and dairy production', Our World In Data, Nov 2019. https://ourworldindata.org/meat-production

3   'Highly pathogenic Asian Avian Influenza A (H5N1) in People, Centers for Disease Control and Prevention, 18 Mar 2015

For Animals

1   Andrew Wasley, Fiona Harvey, Madlen Davies and David Child, 'UK has nearly 800 livestock mega farms, investigation reveals', the *Guardian*, 17 Jul 2017

2   'Farm animals need our help', American Society for the Prevention of Cruelty to Animals website

3   'The Case Against Cages: Evidence in favour of alternative systems for laying hens', RSPCA website

4   'U.S. egg production and hen population', United Egg Producers. https://unitedegg.com/facts-stats/

5   'Layer hen FAQ', RSPCA Australia.

6   Toscano, M.J., et al. 'Explanation for Keel Bone Fractures in Laying Hens: Are There Explanations in Addition to Elevated Egg Production?', *Poultry Science*. 2020; 99 (9): 4183-4194.

7   'At slaughter', Animal Welfare Institute website

8   'Dairy cows fact sheet', Animals Australia website

9   '"A national disgrace": Catalogue of suffering at Scottish abattoirs revealed', Bureau of Investigative Journalism website, 19 Apr 2017

10 'Maternal slaughter at abattoirs: history, causes, cases and the meat industry', *Springer Plus*, 22 Mar 2013

11 'Pregnant cows face slaughter as milk contracts not renewed', Brad Thompson Harvey, *The West Australian*, 1 Oct 2016

12 'Slaughter of pregnant cattle in German abattoirs – current situation and prevalence: a cross-sectional study', *BMC Veterinary Research*, 7 June 2016

13 Singleton, G.H. and Dobson, H., 'A survey of the reasons for culling pregnant cows', *Veterinary Record 136*, 1995

14 'Grazing-based dairying: How the U.S. compares to other countries', Peter van Elzakker, *Progressive Dairyman,* 20 Sept 2013

15 'Pain management issues when castrating and dehorning', Heather Smith Thomas, *Progressive Cattleman*, 25 June 2015

16 'Restaurants drive up cattle slaughter age in quest for more mature beef flavour', Laura Poole, ANB News website, 16 July 2015

17 'How do Canada's welfare standards compete worldwide?', Jennifer Jackson, Farms website, 9 May 2017

18 'Why is nest-building behaviour so important?', FreeFarrowing website

19 'Guidance: caring for pigs', Department for Environment, Food & Rural Affairs, UK Government website, 8 Apr 2013

20 Weary, D.M., and Fraser, D., 'Calling by domestic piglets: reliable signals of need?', *Animal Behaviour*, 1995; 50(4), 1047–1055

21 'The Life of – Pigs', Compassion in World Farming website, 20 May 2013

22 'Handy hints: three ways to manipulate a sheep's breeding cycle', Louise Hartley, *Farmers Guardian*, 8 Oct 2014

23 Kopp, K., et al. 'A Survey of New South Wales Sheep Producer Practices and Perceptions on Lamb Mortality and Ewe Supplementation', Animals. 2020; 10(9):1586. https://www.mdpi.com/2076-2615/10/9/1586

Notes

24 'Lambing Part 4 – ensuring survival of newborn lambs', National Animal Disease Information Service website

25 'Managing newborn lambs', Volac International Limited

26 'Handy hints: three ways to manipulate a sheep's breeding cycle', Louise Hartley, *Farmers Guardian*, 8 Oct 2014

27 'Guidelines on the examination of rams for breeding', Sheep Veterinary Society website, June 2014

28 'Artificial insemination in sheep', Paula I. Menzies, Ontario Veterinary College, University of Guelph, published by Merck & Co

29 'Up to 70 sheep drown in "freak" flash flooding near Llanrwst', Tom Davidson, *Daily Post*, 11 Dec 2015

30 'Sheep guide: a guide to fly strike', That's Farming website, 31 May 2017

31 'Farmers call for help over mounting sheep deaths', Sarah Butler, *Guardian*, 3 Apr 2013

32 Best, C.M., et. al,. 'Sheep farmers' attitudes towards lameness control: Qualitative exploration of factors affecting adoption of the lameness Five-Point Plan', PLoS ONE, 2021; 16(2): e0246798. https://journals.plos.org/plosone/article?id=10.1371/journal.

33 'Lamb', glossary, BBC Good Food website

34 'Managing cull ewes', Agriculture and Horticulture Development Board website, 31 Aug 2016

35 Rob Edwards, 'Farmed salmon deaths from disease reach record high', *The Ferret*, 13 July 2020. https://theferret.scot/farmed-salmon-deaths-disease-reach-record-high/

36 'Unilateral eyestalk ablation', Laboratory of Aquaculture and Artemia Reference Center, Ghent University

37 'Why we need bees: nature's tiny workers put food on our

tables', National Resources Defense Council website, Mar 2011

38 Wheeler, M.M., Robinson, G.E. 'Diet-dependent gene expression in honey bees: Honey vs sucrose or high fructose corn syrup', *Scientific Reports* 4, Article number: 5726 (2014)

For the Environment

1 Olivia Petter, 'Veganism is "single biggest way" to reduce our environmental impact, study finds', *The Independent*, 24 Sept 2020. https://www.independent.co.uk/life-style/health-and-families/veganism-environmental-impact-planet-reduced-plant-based-diet-humans-study-a8378631.html

2 Hannah Ritchie, 'You want to reduce the carbon footprint of your food? Focus on what you eat, not whether your food is local', Our World in Data, 24 Jan 2020. https://ourworldindata.org/food-choice-vs-eating-local

3 G. Myhre., et al. 'Anthropogenic and natural radiative forcing', *Climate Change 2013: The Physical Science Basis. Contribution of working group / report of the Intergovernmental Panel on Climate Change*, 2013

4 'Greenhouse gas emissions', United States Environmental Protection Agency website

5 Helen Harwatt, 'Including animal to plant protein shifts in climate change mitigation policy: a proposed three-step strategy', Climate Policy (2018). 19. 1-9. 10.1080/14693062.2018.1528965. https://www.researchgate.net/publication/329217587_

6 'Do the UN's new numbers for livestock emissions kill the argument for vegetarianism?', Emma Bryce, *Guardian*, 27 Sept 2013

7   'Water scarcity: overview', World Wildlife Fund For Nature website

8   'Water Scarcity', United Nations. https://www.unwater.org/water-facts/scarcity/

9   'The looming threat of water scarcity', Worldwatch Institute website, 19 Mar 2013

10 D'Odorico, P., et. al,. 'The global value of water in agriculture', Proceedings of the National Academy of Sciences Sept 2020, 117 (36) 21985-21993. https://www.pnas.org/content/117/36/21985

11 Bibi van der Zee, 'What is the true cost of eating meat?'. the *Guardian*, 7 May 2018

12 'Cost effective slurry storage strategies on dairy farms', DairyCo, AHDB Dairy website, Feb 2010

13 'Number of cattle worldwide from 2012 to 2017 (in million head)', Statista website, 2017

14 'Pollution from industrialised livestock production', Food and Agriculture Organization website

15 'Toothless Environment Agency is allowing the living world to be wrecked with impunity', George Monbiot, *Guardian,* 12 Nov 2015

16 '10 ways vegetarianism can help save the planet', John Vidal, *Guardian,* 18 Jul 2010

17 Damian Carrington, 'Oceans suffocating as huge dead zones quadruple since 1950, scientists warn', the *Guardian,* 4 Jan 2018

18 '10 ways vegetarianism can help save the planet', John Vidal, *Guardian,* 18 Jul 2010

19 'Environmental and health problems in livestock production: pollution in the food system', The Agribusiness Accountability Initiative

20 'Farming "hotspots" carry air pollution risk, Dutch study finds', Pilita Clark, *Financial Times*, 2 Sept 2016

21 'Forest conversion', World Wildlife Fund for Nature website

22 Alex Lockwood, 'Every meat-eater on the planet is helping to fuel the Amazon forest fires – here's how', *The Independent*, 23 Aug 2019. https://www.independent.co.uk/voices/amazon-forest-fire-brazil-beef-meat-vegan-vegetarian-brazil-a9076236.html

23 'Why soyabeans are the crop of the century', Gregory Meyer, Andres Schipani and Tom Hancock, *Financial Times*, 20 Jun 2017

24 'Amazon deforestation report is major setback for Brazil ahead of climate talks', Jonathan Watts, *Guardian*, 27 Nov 2015

25 "The Sumatran rainforest will mostly disappear within 20 years', John Vidal, *Observer*, 26 May 2013

26 Philip Lymbery, *Dead Zone: Where the Wild Things Were*, Bloomsbury, 2017

27 'The oilpalm connection: is the Sumatran elephant the price of our cheap meat?', Philip Lymbery, *The Ecologist*, 28 Mar 2017

28 'Deforestation and climate change', Greenpeace website

29 'Humanity has wiped out 60% of animal populations since 1970, report finds', Damian Carrington, *The Guardian*, 30 Oct 2018

30 'Most of Amazon rainforest's species extinctions are yet to come', Helen Thompson, *Scientific American*, 13 Jul 2012

31 'Shocking declines in bird numbers show British wildlife is "in serious trouble"', Ian Johnston, *Independent*, 19 May 2017

32 '"Dramatic" decline in European birds linked to industrial agriculture', *Deutsche Welle*, 4 May 2017

33 'The State of Canada's birds 2012', North American Bird Conservation Initiative, Canada, May 2012

34 'Fact check: does Australia have one of the "highest loss of species anywhere in the world?"' ABC News website

35 'Land cover change in Queensland 2014–15', Queensland Government, 2016, p.21

36 'Tree-clearing causing Queensland's greatest animal welfare crisis', World Wildlife Fund for Nature website, 6 Sept 2017

37 'State of Nature 2019', State of Nature Partnerships website

38 'Agriculture and overuse greater threats to wildlife than climate change – study', Jessica Aldred, *Guardian*, 10 Aug 2016

39 Ibid.

40 'If the world adopted a plant-based diet we would reduce global agricultural land use from 4 to 1 billion hectares', Hannah Ritchie, Our World In Data, 4 Mar 2021

41 'Monsters of the oceans: 7 criminal super trawlers that threaten our waters', Greenpeace Australia Pacific, 19 Nov 2014

42 'The boy who stole Queen Victoria's knickers, and 19 other fascinating facts about Buckingham Palace', Soo Kim, *Telegraph*, 7 Apr 2017

43 '5 reasons you should be worried about super trawlers', Animals Australia website, 20 Sept 2017

44 Ibid.

45 '90% of fish stocks are used up – fisheries subsidies must stop', Mukhisa Kituyi, United Nations Conference on Trade and Development, 13 Jul 2018

46 'New paper examines the unintended impact of the EU discard ban', *The Fishing Daily*, 25 Nov 2020.

47 'New US regulations offer better protection from bycatch', *World Wildlife Fund Magazine*, Spring 2017

48 'Maui dolphin', World Wildlife Fund for Nature website

49 'Reducing bycatch of North Atlantic right whales', World Wildlife Fund for Nature website

50 'Bycatch – wasteful and destructive fishing', Greenpeace

51 'Terrible toll of fishing nets on seabirds revealed', Daniel Cressey, *Nature*, 29 May 2013

52 Sandra Laville, 'Dumped fishing gear is biggest plastic polluter in ocean, report finds', the *Guardian*, 6 Nov 2019.

Sustainability and World Hunger

1 'We already grow enough food for 10 billion people – and still can't end hunger', Eric Holtz Gimenez, *Huffington Post*, 2 May 2012

2 'Food', United Nations website

3 '10 ways vegetarianism can help save the planet', John Vidal, Guardian, 18 July 2010

4 'A five-step plan to feed the world', Jonathan Foley, *National Geographic Magazine*, May 2014

5 'World Livestock 2011: Livestock in food security', Food and Agriculture Organization of the United Nations, 2011, p. 21

6 'Livestock – climate change's forgotten sector: global public opinion on meat and dairy consumption', R. Bailey et al., Chatham House, 3 Dec 2014, p. 13

Notes

For Personal Health

1 'The top 10 causes of death', World Health Organization website, Dec 2020

2 Bradbury, K.E. et al, 'Serum concentrations of cholesterol, apolipoprotein A-I and apolipoprotein B in a total of 1694 meat-eaters, fish-eaters, vegetarians and vegans', *European Journal of Clinical Nutrition*, 2014 Feb; 68, 178–183 (February 2014)

3 'Fats explained', British Heart Foundation website

4 'About cholesterol', American Heart Association website

5 Alexander, S. et al., 'A plant-based diet and hypertension', *Journal of Geriatric Cardiology*, 2017; 14(5), 327–330

6 'Adult Obesity Facts', Centers for Disease Control and Prevention, 11 Feb 2021. https://www.cdc.gov/obesity/data/adult.html

7 'Overweight and obesity', Australian Institute of Health and Welfare, 23 July 2020. https://www.aihw.gov.au/reports/australias-health/overweight-and-obesity

8 'Obesity Statistics', House of Commons Library. https://commonslibrary.parliament.uk/research-briefings/sn03336/

9 Tonstad, S., et al., 'Type of Vegetarian Diet, Body Weight, and Prevalence of Type 2 Diabetes', *Diabetes Care*. 2009;32(5), 791–796

10 Benatar, J.R., Stewart, R.A.H., 'Cardiometabolic risk factors in vegans; a meta-analysis of observational studies', PLoS One. 2018 Dec 20;13(12):e0209086. doi: 10.1371/journal.pone.0209086. PMID: 30571724; PMCID: PMC6301673. https://pubmed.ncbi.nlm.nih.gov/30571724/

11 Tuso, P.J., et al., 'Nutritional Update for Physicians: Plant-Based Diets', *The Permanente Journal*. 2013;17(2), 61–66

12 'Obesity is greatest risk factor for type 2 diabetes irrespective of genetics', Mike Watts, Diabetes.co.uk, 19 Apr 2020

13 Michael Greger, *How Not To Die*, Flatiron Books, 2015, p. 106

14 'Ending preventable blindness', Diabetes Australia, 8 Oct 2020.

15 Mike Watts, 'Rising number of disease-related amputations in England', *Diabetes.co.uk*, 27 Feb 2020.

16 Olfert, M.D., Wattick, R.A., 'Vegetarian Diets and the Risk of Diabetes', *Curr Diab Rep.* 2018;18(11):101. Published 2018 Sep 18. doi:10.1007/s11892-018-1070-9. https://www.ncbi.nlm.nih.gov/pmc/articles/PMC6153574/

17 Lee. Y., Park, K. 'Adherence to a vegetarian diet and diabetes risk: a systematic review and meta-analysis of observational studies.' *Nutrients* 2017, 9(6), 603

18 'Vegetarian diets and diabetes', Diabetes UK website

19 'Q&A on the carcinogenicity of the consumption of red meat and processed meat', World Health Organization, Oct 2015

20 Ibid.

21 'Processed meats do cause cancer – WHO', James Gallagher, BBC News website, 26 Oct 2015

22 'Bacon and sausages sales down after cancer scare report', Lexi Finnigan, *Telegraph*, 22 Nov 2015

23 Kizil, M., et al. 'A review on the formation of carcinogenic/mutagenic heterocyclic aromatic amines. *Journal of Food Processing and Technology*, 2:5 (2011)

24 'Chemicals in Meat Cooked at High Temperatures and Cancer Risk', National Cancer Institute, 11 July 2017.

25 'Foodborne illnesses', National Institute of Diabetes and Digestive and Kidney Diseases website

26 Loma Linda University Adventist Health Sciences Center. 'New study associates intake of dairy milk with greater risk of breast cancer: Evidence suggests consistently drinking as little as one cup per day may increase rate of breast cancer up to 50%', ScienceDaily. ScienceDaily, 25 February 2020. https://www.sciencedaily.com/releases/2020/02/200225 101323.htm

27 'On call: diet, testicular cancer, and prostate cancer', Harvard Health Publishing website, Mar 2014

28 Melina, V., et. al., 'Position of the Academy of Nutrition and Dietetics: Vegetarian Diets.' *Journal of the Academy of Nutrition and Dietetics*, 2016 Dec;116(12):1970–1980

For Global Health

1 '10 things you didn't know about bird flu', Michael Greger, *The Ecologist*, 4 Feb 2009

2 'Zoonotic Diseases', Centers for Disease Control and Prevention website

3 'Highly Pathogenic Asian Avian Influenza A (H5N1) in People', Centers for Disease Control and Prevention, 18 Mar 2015. https://www.cdc.gov/flu/avianflu/h5n1-people.htm

4 'Farm animals consume nearly half of all antibiotics', Philip Lymbery, Compassion in World Farming website, 16 Nov 2011

5 'Deadly bird flu strains created by industrial poultry farms', Robert G. Wallace, *The Ecologist*, 30 Jan 2017

6 'Antibiotic-resistant diseases pose "apocalyptic" threat, top expert says', Ian Sample, *The Guardian*, 23 Jan 2013

7 'The drugs don't work - so what will?', James Gallagher, BBC News, 9 Apr 2011

8 'UK on track to cut antibiotic use in animals as total sales drop 9%', Department for Environment, Food & Rural Affairs, UK Government website, 17 Nov 2016

9 'Antibiotic resistance', World Health Organization, 31 Jul 2020. https://www.who.int/news-room/fact-sheets/detail/antibiotic-resistance

10 Princeton University. 'Antibiotic resistance in food animals nearly tripled since 2000', ScienceDaily. ScienceDaily, 9 October 2019. https://www.sciencedaily.com/releases/2019/10/191009132321.htm

11 Ibid.

For the Adventure

1 'A nation of aspiring foodies stuck in a nine-meal rut', Ocado Group website, 22 Feb 2015

The Cheese Addiction

1 'Cheese triggers same part of brain as hard drugs, study finds', Kashmira Gander, *The Independent*, 22 Sept 2020

Nutrition in a Nutshell

1 Nair, R., Maseeh, A. 'Vitamin D: The "sunshine" vitamin', *Journal of Pharmacology & Pharmacotherapeutics.* 2012;3(2): 118-126

2 'Vitamin D deficiency associated with heightened depression, study finds', Ian Johnston, *Independent*, 19 Oct 2016

3 'Iron', National Health Service website

4 'Iron', National Institutes of Health website

5 'Food sources of iron', Dietitians of Canada, 18 Oct 2016

6   Michael Greger, *How Not To Die*, Flatiron Books, 8 Dec 2015, p.71

7   Etemadi, A., 'Mortality from different causes associated with meat, heme iron, nitrates, and nitrites in the NIH-AARP Diet and Health Study: population based cohort study', *BMJ 2017;357:j1957*

8   Zivkovic, A.M., et al., 'Dietary omega-3 fatty acids aid in the modulation of inflammation and metabolic health', *California Agriculture.* 2011;65(3):106-111

9   'Ask the expert: omega-3 fatty acids', Harvard School of Public Health website, 19 June 2007

10 'The vegetarian diet', NHS website

11 'Meet Mungo', *The Washington Post*, 19 Apr 2003

12 'Everything you need to know about vitamin B12 deficiency', Nic Fleming, *Guardian*, 28 Feb 2017

13 'B vitamins and folic acid', NHS website

14 'Vitamin B12: Fact Sheet for Consumers', National Institutes of Health, 7 Jul 2021

15 'Iodine: Food Fact Sheet', The Associations of UK Dietitians. https://www.bda.uk.com/resource/iodine.html

16 Zava, T.T., Zava, D.T., 'Assessment of Japanese iodine intake based on seaweed consumption in Japan: A literature-based analysis', Thyroid Res. 2011;4:14. Published 2011 Oct 5. https://www.ncbi.nlm.nih.gov/pmc/articles/PMC3204293/

17 French, Elizabeth & Mukai, Motoko & Zurakowski, Michael & Rauch, Bradley & Gioia, Gloria & Hillebrandt, Joseph & Henderson, Mark & Schukken, Ynte & Hemling, Thomas. (2016). 'Iodide Residues in Milk Vary between Iodine-Based Teat Disinfectants: Iodine teat disinfectants and milk iodide levels', . . . *Journal of Food Science.* 81. 10.1111/1750-

3841.13358. https://www.researchgate.net/publication/303
796047_Iodide_Residues_in_Milk_Vary_between_Iodine-
Based_Teat_Disinfectants_Iodine_teat_disinfectants_and_
milk_iodide_levels

18 Zava, T.T., Zava, D.T., 'Assessment of Japanese iodine intake
based on seaweed consumption in Japan:
A literature-based analysis', Thyroid Res. 2011;4:14. Published
2011 Oct 5. doi:10.1186/1756-6614-4-14.
https://www.ncbi.nlm.nih.gov/pmc/articles/PMC3204293/

19 Alexander, S., Ostfeld, R.J., Allen, K., Williams, K.A., 'A plant-
based diet and hypertension', J Geriatr Cardiol. 2017;14(5):
327-330. doi:10.11909/j.issn.1671-5411.2017.05.014. https://
www.ncbi.nlm.nih.gov/pmc/articles/PMC5466938/

Vegan Kids

1 'British Dietetic Association confirms well-planned vegan
diets can support healthy living in people of all ages', The
Association of UK Dietitians (formerly British Dietetic
Association), 7 Aug 2017. https://www.bda.uk.com/resource/
british-dietetic-association-confirms-well-planned-vegan-diets-
can-support-healthy-living-in-people-of-all-ages.html

2 Amit, M., 'Vegetarian diets in children and adolescents',
Paediatric Child Health. 2010;15(5):303-314. https://www.ncbi.
nlm.nih.gov/pmc/articles/PMC2912628/

3 Baroni, L., Goggi, S., Battaglino, R., Berveglieri, M., Fasan, I.,
Filippin, D., Griffith, P., Rizzo, G., Tomasini, C., Tosatti, M.A.,
Battino, M.A., 'Vegan Nutrition for Mothers and Children:
Practical Tools for Healthcare Providers', *Nutrients*. 2019;
11(1):5. https://www.mdpi.com/2072-6643/11/1/5/htm

4 Sebastiani, G., Herranz Barbero, A., Borrás-Novell, C., et al.,

'The Effects of Vegetarian and Vegan Diet during Pregnancy on the Health of Mothers and Offspring', *Nutrients*. 2019;11(3):557. Published 2019 Mar 6. doi:10.3390/nu11030557. https://www.ncbi.nlm.nih.gov/pmc/articles/PMC6470702/

5   'Weight management before, during and after pregnancy', National Institute for Health and Care Excellence, 28 Jul 2020. https://www.nice.org.uk/guidance/ph27/chapter/Recommendations

6   Baroni, L., Goggi, S., Battaglino, R., Berveglieri, M., Fasan, I., Filippin, D., Griffith, P., Rizzo, G., Tomasini, C., Tosatti, M.A., Battino, M.A.. 'Vegan Nutrition for Mothers and Children: Practical Tools for Healthcare Providers', *Nutrients*. 2019; 11(1):5. https://www.mdpi.com/2072-6643/11/1/5/htm

7   'Have a healthy diet in pregnancy', National Health Service. https://www.nhs.uk/pregnancy/keeping-well/have-a-healthy-diet/

8   'Pregnancy and pre-conception', British Nutrition Foundation. https://www.nutrition.org.uk/nutritionscience/life/pregnancy-and-pre-conception.html?start=5

9   Sebastiani, G., Herranz Barbero, A., Borrás-Novell, C., et al., 'The Effects of Vegetarian and Vegan Diet during Pregnancy on the Health of Mothers and Offspring', *Nutrients*. 2019;11(3):557. Published 2019 Mar 6. doi:10.3390/nu11030557. https://www.ncbi.nlm.nih.gov/pmc/articles/PMC6470702/

10 Angela V Saunders, Winston J Craig and Surinder K Baines. 'Zinc and Vegetarian Diets'. *Med J Aust* 2013; 199 (4): S17-S21 https://www.mja.com.au/journal/2013/199/4/zinc-and-vegetarian-diets

11 Sebastiani, G., Herranz Barbero, A., Borrás-Novell, C., et al., 'The Effects of Vegetarian and Vegan Diet during Pregnancy on the Health of Mothers and Offspring', *Nutrients*. 2019;11(3):557. Published 2019 Mar 6. doi:10.3390/nu11030557. https://www.ncbi.nlm.nih.gov/pmc/articles/PMC6470702/

12 'Have a healthy diet in pregnancy', National Health Service. https://www.nhs.uk/pregnancy/keeping-well/have-a-healthy-diet/

13 'B vitamins and folic acid', National Health Service. https://www.nhs.uk/conditions/vitamins-and-minerals/vitamin-b/

14 'Vitamin D in Pregnancy', Royal College of Obstetricians & Gynaecologists, June 2014. https://www.rcog.org.uk/globalassets/documents/guidelines/scientific-impact-papers/vitamin_d_sip43_june14.pdf

15 'Foods to avoid in pregnancy', National Health Service. https://www.nhs.uk/pregnancy/keeping-well/foods-to-avoid/

16 'Vegetarian or vegan and pregnant', National Health Service. https://www.nhs.uk/live-well/eat-well/vegetarian-and-vegan-mums-to-be/

17 'SMA Wysoy Soya Infant Formula', SMA. https://www.smababy.co.uk/formula-milk/wysoy-infant-formula/

18 Claire McCarthy MD, 'What parents need to know about a vegan diet', Harvard Health Publishing. 7 Jan 2020. https://www.health.harvard.edu/blog/what-parents-need-to-know-about-a-vegan-diet-2020010718625

19 Ibid.

20 Amit, M., 'Vegetarian diets in children and adolescents', *Paediatric Child Health.* 2010;15(5):303-314. https://www.ncbi.nlm.nih.gov/pmc/articles/PMC2912628/

21 Sutter, Daniel. (2017), 'The impact of vegan diet on health and growth of children and adolescents – Literature review', 10.13140/RG.2.2.30001.68963. https://www.researchgate.net/publication/318135128_

22 Amit, M., 'Vegetarian diets in children and adolescents', *Paediatric Child Health*. 2010;15(5):303-314. https://www.ncbi.nlm.nih.gov/pmc/articles/PMC2912628/

23 Menal-Puey, S., Martínez-Biarge, M., Marques-Lopes, I., 'Developing a Food Exchange System for Meal Planning in Vegan Children and Adolescents', *Nutrients*. 2019; 11(1):43. https://www.mdpi.com/2072-6643/11/1/43

24 Baroni, L., Goggi, S., Battaglino, R., Berveglieri, M., Fasan, I., Filippin, D., Griffith, P., Rizzo, G., Tomasini, C., Tosatti, M.A., Battino, M.A.. 'Vegan Nutrition for Mothers and Children: Practical Tools for Healthcare Providers', Nutrients. 2019; 11(1):5. https://www.mdpi.com/2072-6643/11/1/5/htm

Vegan Myths

1 '10 ways vegetarianism can help save the planet', John Vidal, *Guardian*, 18 July 2010

2 Olivia Petter, 'Veganism is the "single biggest way" to reduce our environmental impact study finds', *The Independent*, 24 Sept 2020. https://www.independent.co.uk/life-style/health-and-families/veganism-environmental-impact-planet-reduced-plant-based-diet-humansstudy-a8378631.html

3 'Antibiotic Overuse in Livestock Farming', Alliance to Save our Antibiotics. https://www.saveourantibiotics.org/the-issue/antibiotic-overuse-in-livestock-farming/

4 'Zoonotic Diseases', Centers for Diseae Control and Prevention. https://www.cdc.gov/onehealth/basics/zoonotic-diseases.html

5   'Veganism is the "single biggest way" to reduce our
    environmental impact study finds, Olivia Petter, *The
    Independent*, 24 Sept 2020

6   'Lambing to order!', Tim Tyne, Country Smallholding, 6 May
    2014

7   'Amazon rainforest's final frontier under threat from oil and
    soya', John Vidal, *Guardian*, 16 Feb 2017

8   'How can we stop using soya linked to deforestation?' Tom
    Levitt, *The Guardian*, 25 Nov 2020

9   'Soy is everywhere', World Wide Fund for Nature website

10 Ibid.